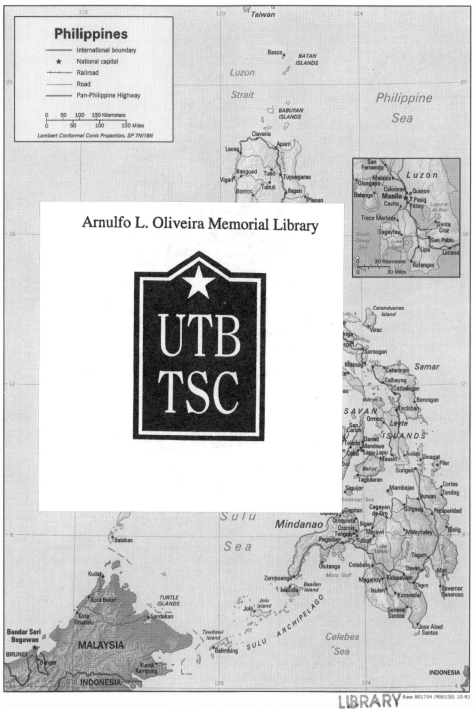

All This Hell

All This

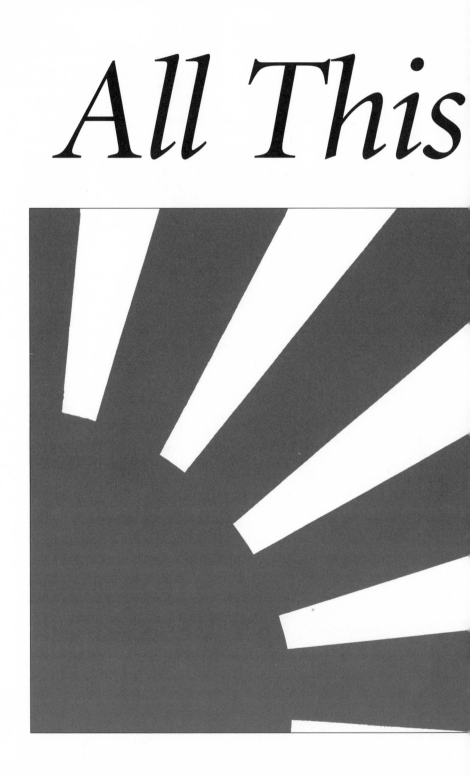

Hell

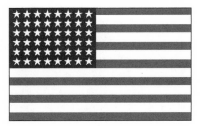

U.S. Nurses
Imprisoned
by the
Japanese

Evelyn M.
Monahan
and
Rosemary
Neidel-Greenlee

THE UNIVERSITY
PRESS OF KENTUCKY

Publication of this volume was made possible in part by a grant from the National Endowment for the Humanities.

Scholarly publisher for the Commonwealth,
serving Bellarmine College, Berea College, Centre
College of Kentucky, Eastern Kentucky University,
The Filson Club Historical Society, Georgetown College,
Kentucky Historical Society, Kentucky State University,
Morehead State University, Murray State University,
Northern Kentucky University, Transylvania University,
University of Kentucky, University of Louisville,
and Western Kentucky University.

Editorial and Sales Offices: The University Press of Kentucky
663 South Limestone Street, Lexington, Kentucky 40508-4008

04 03 02 01   3 4 5

Library of Congress Cataloging-in-Publication Data

All this hell / Evelyn Monahan and Rosemary Neidel-Greenlee.
        p.   cm.
        ISBN 0-8131-2148-5 (alk. paper)
    1. World War, 1939-1945—Prisoners and prisons, Japanese.
2. Nurses—United States—History—20th century. 3. World War,
1939-1945—Medical care—United States. 4. Prisoners of war—
Philippines—History—20th century. 5. Prisoners of war—
Japan—History—20th century. I. Monahan, Evelyn.
        II. Neidel-Greenlee, Rosemary, 1941– .
    D805.P6 A433 2000
    940.54'7252'09599—dc21   99-045226

Manufactured in the United States of America

Memory is the mother of all wisdom.

Aeschlyus, *Prometheus Bound*

Contents

Illustrations follow pages 20, 84, and 164.

Preface

This book had its origins early in 1988, when, at the beginning of an interview, a former prisoner of war (POW) nurse asked, "Do you really want to hear this?" The answer was a firm, "Absolutely!" This exchange began more than a decade of research into the history and experiences of eighty-four military nurses who were prisoners of the Japanese during World War II.

From this first interview, we knew that we were in a race with time. Many of these women spoke of friends and comrades who had died in recent years and of the dwindling number of Christmas cards that arrived each season. They also expressed fear that after they too were gone, no one would care about their service to their country. All in one way or another asked, "Who will remember?"

Thoughtful deliberation of that inquiry led to truths that were hard to accept and difficult to understand. At the top of the list was that former POW army nurses were discouraged from talking about their combat and POW experiences even to their families. At redistribution centers and in reorientation programs, the POW experience was presented to these women as a stigma and they were told that it was time for them to become "ladies" again. This admonition joined with their natural reluctance to tell their stories to form a psychological alloy stronger than steel. In addition, military history and the history of war have traditionally been treated as a male domain, which is another reason these women's deeds did not make it into many history books. After their individual hometowns welcomed many of these nurses on their return, their accomplishments as members of the Army and Navy Nurse Corps faded rapidly from the American memory.

As we continued our research, we were delighted to discover that we owed a large debt of gratitude to a small group of people who acted in late 1982 and early 1983 to bring recognition to these women and preserve some of their experiences. Sam Moody, founder of the American Defenders of Bataan and Corregidor and a member of the Veterans Administration Advisory Committee for Former Prisoners of War, pointed out that some former POWs were military nurses. Dorothy Starbuck, a Women's Army Corps veteran who served in the European theater during World War II, was at that time chief benefits director of the Veterans Administration (VA). She acted on Moody's information immediately and wrote to some of the former POW military nurses in late December 1982. Before the end of January 1983, the women responded and provided addresses and married names for other former POW nurses. Through Starbuck's instigation and with the sponsorship and financial support of many, including veterans' service organizations and VA employee groups, the former POWs were brought to Washington, D.C., in April 1983 for three days of activities and recognition. The women were received and addressed by President Ronald Reagan in the Oval Office, and each was interviewed for the Army Nurse Corps Oral History program. In addition, the Veterans Administration and the Department of Defense cooperated in producing a twenty-eight-minute documentary video, *We All Came Home*, which includes portions of personal interviews with several of these women and archival footage of prison camp liberation in 1945. Unfortunately, few people have seen the video and even fewer know about what these women did for their country.

In a time when heroes are often defined by the number of "runs batted in" or "yards gained rushing," these heroic women stand in timeless contrast to society's shifting values. The standards reached and surpassed by each of these former POWs have always been the bedrock from which and on which freedom's national heroes are born and endure. Each of these women transcended what is expected of any soldier and reached what might be hoped for from the bravest. All of the former POW military women conducted themselves in the finest traditions of the armed forces and their chosen profession, and they became living examples of what our country may expect and hope for from its military women. In short, they earned the title of national heroes. And what can we learn from these heroes? They teach by example that freedom is not free and that Americans, male and female, have always been willing to risk everything for the right to be free.

As the twentieth century draws to a close, historical accuracy and justice demand that what these nurses endured and the spirit in which they bore their burdens should be recognized by the American people who share in the gift of freedom these veterans helped purchase.

We are honored to have known these heroines of the "Other Alamo," these "Angels of Bataan and Corregidor," and privileged to be one small link in passing their legacy on to future generations.

A very special thank-you to our friends Hannah Branton, Lisa Lowden, and Adam Langley for their technical assistance and support.

1

Pacific Paradise

We were young then and we didn't think too much about it.
My father told me, "Don't go; there's going to be a war." But
when you're young, you just don't think about that. When
you have somewhere to go, the thing is to go.

Lt. Col. Eunice Young, USAF (Ret.)

Through the 1930s and until the last month of 1941, American army nurses waited on a long list of volunteers for assignments to the Philippine Islands. For navy nurses it was the "luck of the draw" that brought them to the Pacific paradise, where short duty hours allowed them to spend bright tropical days swimming and playing golf. News from nurses who had completed their two-year tour and returned to the United States resulted in a seemingly endless supply of military nurses hoping to serve in the storybook culture of the tropics.

Long years of the Depression in the United States led many young graduate nurses to join the Army and Navy Nurse Corps. Military nursing looked like a good opportunity for those confronting a sparse civilian market that paid nurses on average two dollars a day, if they were fortunate enough to find employment. Nursing duties in civilian hospitals were performed mainly by unpaid student nurses, who, once they were graduated, would find the world of private duty nursing seriously restricted by the ability of individuals to purchase their services. Nursing journals carried advertisements for the Army and Navy Nurse Corps. Young women who were adventurous enough to enter the field of nursing, which many parents and others did not consider a ladylike occupation, found it even more daring to enlist in the military nurse corps, which promised comparatively good salaries, a chance to serve one's country, travel to distant places, and possible contact with cultures few civilian women would ever see. It is more than fair to argue that only the most brave young women joined the Army and Navy Nurse Corps and that only the most adventurous among these volunteered to serve in the Philippines, a group of tropical islands on the other side of the world and only hours away from Japan by air.

Even if one believed that war between Japan and the United States was inevitable, there was no knowing when and where such a war might begin. War Plan Orange 3, a strategy to defend the Philippines in the event of war with Japan, was known to a select group in the War Department and to Gen. Douglas MacArthur and his top commanders in the Philippines. No one in the Army and Navy Nurse Corps had ever heard of War Plan Orange 3. Given their youth and their spirit of adventure and the strong belief of most young people in their own indestructibility, it is doubtful that the disclosure of the war plan would have influenced these nurses in their willingness to serve in the Philippines. After all, even General MacArthur, who had been recalled to active duty on 26 July 1941 and placed in charge of the Allied Forces Philippine Command, believed that if war broke out between the United States and Japan, it would not be before April 1942.

There were signs of uneasiness that military nurses in or on their way to the Philippine Islands might have heeded, but the invincibility felt by the young, combined with the powerful defense of denial, let them pass many warning signs with little notice. Two of these signs involved the Army Nurse Corps directly. On 8 September 1939, a state of limited emergency was proclaimed as a result of the war declared in Europe five days earlier. At the time, 625 regular army nurses were on active duty. The authorized strength of the regulars in the Army Nurse Corps was raised to 949. On 30

June 1940, 15,770 nurses enrolled in the First Reserve of the American Red Cross Nursing Service and were considered available for active service whenever they were needed.

In late winter 1940, the War Department ordered that the dependents of all military personnel in the Philippines be evacuated to the United States. Navy dependents sailed for home in March 1941, followed in May by army dependents. The last ship to carry dependents away from the Philippines was the USS *Washington,* which sailed on 14 May 1941.

The number of ships leaving the United States for the Philippines increased dramatically. Military personnel and supplies, which customarily arrived by ship once every three months, now steamed into the harbor once or twice each month. Most of these vessels docking in Manila Harbor delivered army nurses to begin their two-year tours in what they expected would be a tropical Eden.

Military nurses received 50 percent of the pay of male officers of the same rank. A nurse with the relative rank of second lieutenant earned $88.60 a month. Of that amount, $70.00 was base pay, and $18.60 was a subsistence allowance. Minnie Breese, a native of Arlington Heights, Illinois, reflected the feelings of many army nurses when she said, "My first duty station was Fort Riley, Kansas. My mother took me to the train and asked, 'How much are they going to pay you?' I said, 'I don't know. I never asked them. I'll get room and board.' That's all I cared about—and a job."[1]

Despite warnings from family members that war with Japan was likely, nurses counted themselves lucky to be the recipients of a plum assignment to the Philippines. Lt. Anna E. Williams, a native of Harrisburg, Pennsylvania, was very young when she explained to her family why she had volunteered for duty there. Williams said, "When I told my parents, well, you know at that age you don't ever think your family knows very much about what is happening in the world . . . I was just 21 . . . and Mother said, 'Ann Eleanor, why are you going to the Philippines? War is starting there. There's going to be a war and it's going to start in the Philippine area.' I said, 'Oh, Mother, come on.' Thinking . . . she doesn't know—

I don't know what winds she was reading, but anyway, I said, 'Mother, look, I am an Army nurse and that's ... [where] I want to be. If there's a war, I should be there working.' "[2]

Relative rank did not confer a military title, and all army and navy nurses were addressed as "Miss." The young women went directly from civilian life to work in military hospitals without the benefit of military training or even a military orientation. The army nurses were provided with six white duty uniforms distinguished from a civilian nurse's uniform only by the military insignia they were required to wear on their collars. Neither their relative rank nor the insignia they wore entitled them to the salute required by male officers.

When army nurses disembarked from transport ships in Manila Harbor, they were welcomed by an army band. They walked down the gangplank wearing high heels, chiffon dresses, picture hats, and white gloves. They looked more like debutantes arriving for a social occasion than military nurses reporting for duty. Instead of khaki uniforms, their luggage contained long dresses for dinner and any post activities after 1800 and party dresses for special occasions. The formality of the islands had an air of elegance to twenty-two-year-old Lieutenant Earlyn Black, who joined the Army Nurse Corps in 1940. Lt. Black recalled those days: "Each evening we dressed for dinner in long dresses. The men dressed in tuxedos, dinner jackets with the cummerbunds. It was very formal type living. Even to go to the movies, we'd put on a long dress."[3]

The weather was so hot and humid that nurses were not required to wear stockings on duty. Except for the rainy season, which began in late May and continued through July, every day looked like postcard-colored tropics. The fragrance of gardenias and honeysuckle permeated the humid air so thoroughly that one could almost taste it.

There were five army hospitals and one navy hospital in the Philippines before the Japanese attack on Pearl Harbor. The number of army nurses stationed at those hospitals doubled in the last six months of 1941. In addition to the requirement of completing two years of military service in the United States, each nurse assigned to the Philippines had to be in perfect health. Because transports arrived only once every three months with supplies and replacements, the nursing staff was shorthanded for quite a while when a nurse became too ill to continue working. Tuberculosis was feared everywhere, but nowhere more than in the Philippines. If TB infected one's lungs in that tropical climate, it progressed with lightning rapidity. Heat and humidity acted as incubators for disease and infection even in that prewar paradise.

Duty hours for the nurses varied slightly, according to where they were stationed; however, the leave policy for all medical personnel throughout the Philippine Command was the same. They frequently used accrued leave when returning to the United States after completing their tour, visiting China and Japan or India and Europe on their way home. This opportunity to see countries few U.S. civilians visited in those days was one more attraction of a Philippine tour of service.

While in the islands, medical personnel were placed on ten or fourteen days of "detached service" for visits to the southern islands or Baguio. Camp John Hay on the outskirts of Baguio was approximately two hundred miles north of Manila and at least ten degrees cooler than the rest of the Philippines. Baguio, three miles from the camp, had many open-air markets that sold handmade crafts to the tourists who made their way to its picturesque and cool streets. At an elevation of 5,029 feet, Camp John Hay seemed to its military visitors more like a mountain resort than an army post.

Nurses were able to visit the various station hospitals and Manila on weekends or days off. The nurses' quarters maintained extra beds to accommodate visiting nurses. The six army hospitals on Luzon and Corregidor were distinguished by location, size, and types of patients treated. Nurses' quarters were essentially equivalent in the amenities they offered their residents, but their physical structure differed in accordance with their location and the size of the nursing staff.

Sternberg General Hospital consisted of a two-story building that, in the style of Spanish architecture, stood around an enclosed courtyard. It was located at a busy intersection in downtown Manila, within walking distance of the municipal golf and tennis courts, the old walled city, an up-to-date shopping area, and the Army and Navy Club. The hospital was surrounded by city noises: traffic, police, and fire sirens and the shrill screams of ambulances delivering the sick and injured for medical care to Sternberg and civilian hospitals.

Until the last half of 1941, the Sternberg, as it was called by most of its staff, had approximately 450 beds, between fifteen and twenty nurses, a large laboratory section for research on tropical diseases, a barrio ward that treated Filipinos, an officers' ward, an enlisted ward, a score of private rooms, the usual operating suites, x-ray equipment, and the services of a civilian physiotherapist and a dietitian. Before the Japanese attack on Pearl Harbor, the relatively small patient load allowed time for numerous medical research projects.

Because of the tropical heat and humidity of Manila, nurses on day shifts worked an average of four hours a day, with the afternoon shift beginning at 1230. The night shifts worked eight hours and faced the difficulty of trying to sleep in the heat of the day. Shifts were rotated to afford equality of duty hours.

As a general hospital, the Sternberg received cases too complicated for the smaller station hospitals and all psychiatric cases. The Sternberg was reportedly the best-equipped hospital in the Philippines; however, nurses who transferred there directly from Walter Reed General Hospital in Washington, D.C., found it wanting in equipment and timeliness in serving patients. Lt. Anna Williams had a particularly disturbing experience there. "I was quite upset because one of my patients had a heart attack. I called for the doctor and also called for an oxygen tent.... Everything was so slow coming that the patient died before—I ... [got] ... the oxygen tent."[4]

Because of the lack of refrigeration and poor health practices in the city, there were few places where army nurses were permitted to eat off the post. The chief nurse did, however, encourage the nurses to learn about Philippine culture and customs. Most nurses followed the suggestion gladly and visited agricultural sites, tobacco farms, hat factories, and other local points of interest.

The culture and customs of the military were also a part of the nurses' experience and sometimes affected their workload. On the night of a military payday, the number of patients at the Sternberg increased predictably. Lt. Madeline Ullom, a twenty-nine-year-old nurse from O'Neill, Nebraska, remembered those nights vividly: "We had the other components of the Army nearby, and also Cavite Navy Base was only about nine miles away. So lots of times on payday night the men went down to the Pink Poodle or some of those places, and about 2:00 AM, you got in accidents where somebody got into [a] fight, and they got slashed up a bit."[5]

The four other army hospitals on Luzon had nurses' quarters consisting of wooden bungalows that housed three or four nurses in private rooms with a shared bath and a common living area. Kitchen and dining facilities were in the chief nurses' bungalows where nurses gathered for meals. As a defense against insects and to take advantage of every passing breeze, the bungalows were built on stilts and had screened-in windows and porches. Every closet had its own electric light to help cut down on mildew caused by high humidity. Nurses had few if any chores outside duty hours because each nursing staff had its own cook, laundresses, and houseboys.

Fort McKinley was approximately seven miles from Manila. It had been a dispensary for Filipino Scouts before the last six months of 1941, when the Army Medical Department converted it into a 250–bed hospital. The newly appointed chief nurse for this facility, Eleanor O'Neill, a forty-two-year-old native of Providence, Rhode Island, who held the relative rank of first lieutenant, transferred there from Fort Stotsenberg. She faced the immense job of converting the dispensary into a large hospital. Army nurses were gradually added to Lieutenant O'Neill's staff as the hospital began to take shape, but the nurses' quarters and messing facilities were never able to accommodate the growing number of nurses assigned there.

Nurses' duty hours were split because of the tropical climate. The split shift ran from 0700 to 0900 and then from 1300 until 1900. The four-hour day shift ran from 0900 to 1300. The night shift worked from 1900 until 0700.

Lt. Hattie R. Brantley, a twenty-five-year-old nurse from Jefferson, Texas, spoke of conversations during meals at Fort McKinley when thoughts of war were masked by denial and humor. "The general feeling among the nurses was that there was no possibility of war with Japan. It was a joke and our Chief Nurse would say in the nurses' mess, 'Have another biscuit, girls. You're going to need this when the Japs get us.' Well, we'd all laugh. They started sending dependents back and there were few when I got there in June 1941. It should have been evident to everybody that we were getting ready for something, but we just sort of rocked along and were happy, and didn't give it too much thought. But Peg O'Neill would say, 'Have another biscuit, girls,' and believe me, after we got to prison, we thought about those biscuits we didn't eat."[6]

In conversations with the army pilots from nearby Clark Field, the Fort Stotsenberg nurses learned of signs of war, but as twenty-two-year-old Lt. Rita Palmer said: "We were just kids and we were in a strange and different country. We were excited by everything we did. I remember being told by pilots that they were flying into formations of Japanese planes, and they were concerned. They tried to report it, but no one listened. But I don't think . . . we gave it a second thought."[7]

The flourishing social life on post was another deterrent to serious thoughts of war. Nurses would visit Baguio when they could on weekends. Every Sunday the Officers' Club would hold a special affair at which the general and other senior officers served hot dogs, hamburgers, and beer to junior officers and nurses.

Fort Stotsenberg was approximately seventy miles north of Manila. It had been a cavalry post in earlier days, and polo matches were held there. Clark Field was adjacent to Stotsenberg, and pilots and nurses visited back and forth regularly. Approximately six nurses and one chief nurse were stationed at Stotsenberg.

Nurses frequently were invited to dinner in the officers' quarters. Four male officers shared a house, a Chinese cook, a houseboy, and two or three other servants. Male officers wore white dinner jackets and bow ties. When going out to dinner or a bridge game at the officers' quarters in the rainy season, nurses carried their shoes and often waded through several inches of water to reach their transportation. When they arrived at their destination, their host would hand them a towel to dry their feet, and they would sit and put on their shoes. During the rainy season in the Philippines, it was as customary as your host taking your coat and hanging it in the hall closet, and nurses acclimated to it as they did to other customs in the islands.

The station hospital at Camp John Hay near Baguio had between thirty and thirty-five beds and a nursing staff of two army nurses, both with the relative rank of second lieutenant. One of those nurses, Lt. Beatrice E. Chambers, the daughter of a British mother and an American father, a veteran of the Spanish-American War, had been born and raised in the Baguio area. She had attended nursing school in the United States and joined the Army Nurse Corps before being stationed at Camp John Hay.

Fort Mills was located on Corregidor, commonly known as the Rock, a fortress at the mouth of Manila Bay. The quartermaster provided boat transportation to and from Manila once every day. The one-way trip took two and a half hours.

Fort Mills was built on the three natural levels of Corregidor. The hospital with approximately two hundred beds was located on Topside, as was the enlisted barracks, the longest military barracks in the world. The nurses' quarters were located at Middleside, and nurses either rode a streetcar, which the quartermaster ran every thirty minutes, or climbed the one hundred concrete steps that connected Topside and Middleside. At Bottomside was the barrio, the native village, and the entrances to Malinta Tunnel.

The nurses' quarters consisted of two large houses originally used as living quarters for the families of male officers. The front of the quarters faced Manila Bay. At night the lights of Manila could be seen from the two buildings. The ten to twelve nurses stationed at Fort Mills had private rooms with connecting baths. The chief nurse had a suite next to the common dining room. She was in charge of the nurses' mess and supervised a Chinese cook and his helper.

The beautiful setting of Fort Mills was enhanced by the large numbers of gardenias, honeysuckle, and other tropical vegetation. In the isolation of Corregidor there were no mosquitoes or street and traffic noises throughout the night, but instead the sounds of crickets to lull one to sleep. This situation worked in reverse for many of the nurses based at the Sternberg or the Manila area who visited Fort Mills. The silence and the crickets kept them awake.

Fort Mills had a well-stocked commissary and three post exchanges that provided almost anything a shopper might wish to purchase. The fort also had two theaters, tennis courts, swim clubs, a golf course, a bowling alley, and an Officers' Club. Since Corregidor was isolated and relatively small, military personnel socialized with each other. To one degree or another, this was true of all military personnel stationed in the Philippines. In a sense, they became family to each other, a close-knit community that worked and played together. The split shifts worked by nurses on the day shifts allowed them more time to take advantage of Fort Mills's amenities.

After the navy evacuated its military dependents in March 1941 and the army followed in May, married officers were invited to the nurses' quarters for dinner on a regular rotation basis at Fort Mills. The army nurses were the only women left on Corregidor until several Filipina nurses were hired in late 1941, when nursing staffs were being augmented everywhere in the Philippine Command.

The Canacao Naval Hospital was located at the base of Cavite Peninsula. A radio station was on the west end of the hospital, and the facility itself faced Canacao Bay, directly across from the Cavite

Navy Yard. The yard was only half a mile from the naval hospital. Transportation from Cavite to Manila was provided by a ferry that ran on a regular timetable.

The twelve navy nurses who were assigned to the 150–bed naval hospital lived in a two-story nurses' quarters that had wide screened-in verandas on each level. Houseboys kept the floors polished and the brightwork shining. Nurses worked an eight-hour day and had every third weekend off. A full social life was available at the Cavite Officers' Club and the Army and Navy Club in Manila.

Unlike army nurses, in the spring of 1941 the navy nurses were advised that outgoing mail was being censored and were instructed to send home valuables and souvenirs. The naval command saw a fast-approaching military emergency. Thirty-one-year-old Lt. Edwina Todd from Pomona, California, remembered her time at Canacao before America entered the war: "By September the fleet was rarely in port, practice blackouts were frequent. Thus we had adequate warning to prepare for the emergency. Consequently extra medical supplies had been ordered from the States; however, these failed to arrive in time. We did have a chance to do the most with what we had. Hundreds of surgical dressings of all sizes were made and sterilized. Nurses were asked to order anything they needed to prepare their wards for casualties. Thus all wards were equipped with surgical instruments, suture material, dressings, adhesive, bandages, bandage scissors, normal saline solution, extra blankets, plasma, N.S.S. and I.V. intravenous sets."[8]

Although the island of Guam is approximately fifteen hundred miles from the Philippines, it was of major strategic importance in Japan's opening attack against America. The navy nurses stationed on Guam would be the first American military women to be taken prisoners of war by the Japanese.

The naval hospital on Guam was small and staffed by five military nurses. After a year at this duty station, nurses were frequently transferred to Canacao, and so navy nurses at both hospitals often served together.

Guam was in some ways a microcosm of Corregidor, without Malinta hill or tunnel. Like the Rock, Guam was isolated, and its military personnel worked and played together. The recreational activities enjoyed on the island included swimming, sailing, deep-sea fishing, golf, badminton, and tennis. A bridge club met every Tuesday, there was a dance once a month at the Officers' Club, and the occasional cocktail party filled in the time in between.

Navy nurses on Guam seemed to have a more realistic view than those in the Philippines of the approaching war with Japan. Lt. Leona Jackson, a thirty-two-year-old native of Union, Ohio, spoke of her days on Guam before Pearl Harbor: "We were five years too late in trying to fortify anything out there [U.S.-controlled south Pacific islands]. . . .There were no fortifications on Guam whatsoever. . . .We would be sitting ducks if the Japs came there and I fully felt that they would. As soon as I knew that the fortification was going on in the Marianas [the island group to which Guam belongs], I felt that they were preparing for war."[9]

Although individual nurses in the Philippines were unaware that preparations for war were taking place in the last half of 1941, they were affected by some of the resulting changes. The pressures of converting a dispensary into a hospital with all its attendant problems and the obsolete and inadequate equipment the army provided probably contributed to the heart attack suffered by Chief Nurse Eleanor O'Neill in 1941. She was temporarily replaced by Lt. Clara Mueller.

Other changes also affected the nursing staff. Miss E. Valine Messner, the chief nurse of the Philippine Command, was rotated back to the United States and was replaced by fifty-six-year-old Maude C. Davison, who held the relative rank of captain. Captain Davison, who was born in Canada on 27 March 1885 and chose to become an American citizen, joined the Army Nurse Corps in 1918. Her leadership would be essential in the months to come and would mean life or death for her nurses in the approaching war and their imprisonment.

The military was moving increasing numbers of soldiers, sailors, and medical personnel westward into the Pacific. In April 1941, Bertha Evans, a thirty-seven-year-old native of Oregon and a nine-year veteran of the Navy Nurse Corps, took her orders for Canacao and boarded the USS *Henderson* in San Francisco for a thirty-day voyage to Manila. She described a portion of that leisurely thirteen-knots-an-hour voyage:

> It was the slowest thing that you ever were on. But I enjoyed it. Of course, we were filled with sailors going to Honolulu to meet the fleet. And we had Army officers aboard too. And that's where I learned about all the prospects of war. On the east coast there was not a word said about it. It was very quiet. They just didn't talk about it. I remember asking at the Bureau whether I should take all my gear out there. "Certainly. Make yourself comfortable. You have nice quarters and all that." And I did it to my sorrow. . . .
>
> On the way to Honolulu, I met some reserve officers that were called to active duty. One of them said to Helen Gorzelanski, the nurse I was traveling with, that he felt sorry [for] us girls. He said, "You'll be eating fish heads and rice before you come home." I said, "Do you really think so?" And he said, "I know so." Then I started to wonder whether we were really going to be in a war.
>
> We stopped [at Midway] and they took us ashore to show us the installations. We saw the famous gooney birds and saw all the water towers up in the air. The Army officers aboard the ship said, "That shows you that civilians are taking care of this. They wouldn't listen to us. The first thing the enemy would knock out in case of a war would be your water supply."
>
> We didn't actually go ashore in Guam because we had measles aboard. The inhabitants of Guam were not inoculated and they didn't want to have a plague start there and kill them all. . . .
>
> When we arrived in Manila, the World War I fleet was

there.... That's all they had out there! I thought Oh my
God! If we have a war we're sunk....

But I didn't dwell on that. I just had a real nice time.
The nurses were all very cordial.... Life went on and we
had nice cocktail parties at the club and I liked my duty.[10]

The last two convoys carrying military nurses to the Philippines left San Francisco on 26 September and 24 October 1941.
The October convoy was the first silent sailing from this port. Previously, sailings were announced in the newspapers, and someone
finally decided that that gave the Germans and the Japanese more
information than the American government wished them to know.
So following the departure of the USS *Holbrook,* which left in September, the USS *Scott* and the USS *Coolidge* left for the Philippine
Islands without a public announcement. Twelve army nurses traveled on the *Scott* and twelve on the *Coolidge.* Among the other passengers were the men of a tank unit with their tanks and
maintenance equipment. Each ship also carried air corps officers.
When the ships reached Honolulu, no troops were allowed to go
ashore. Lt. Phyllis Arnold, a slim, five-foot, four-inch, twenty-five-
year-old from Minneapolis, Minnesota, particularly remembered
the voyage from Honolulu to Manila.

When we left Honolulu, we began to realize that things
were serious. There was a destroyer on each side of us.
Every so often a flight of airplanes accompanied us. We
hit Guam and we couldn't go into the harbor. We had to
be taken in on launches because the harbor was mined
.... All this, the destroyers on the side, the airplanes, and
the mined harbor should have told me we were getting
ready for war. Another thing happened. In Honolulu, the
troops weren't allowed to go ashore. They [those in
command] said that they had been exposed to something, and that they couldn't go ashore because they
might contaminate [someone or something].... The
closer we got to the Philippines, [the more] I should have

realized how serious it was, but at that time I was [a] very slap-happy person. I loved to dance, I enjoyed being a good nurse, but when I was off duty, I either danced, played golf, tennis or went swimming.[11]

The *Holbrook* disembarked its nurses six weeks before the Japanese attack on Hawaii. The *Scott* and the *Coolidge* arrived in Manila Bay on 28 November 1941. Time was closing in fast on the Pacific paradise, yet for those nurses stationed in the Philippines before 7 December 1941, the hell of war that was about to descend upon them was unimaginable.

2

Paradise Lost

Unprepared is the word that describes us best. . . . The handwriting was on the wall, but nobody read it.
Lt. Col. Hattie R. Brantley, USA, NC (Ret.)

Military nurses in the Philippines awakened to news that would change the world forever. Radios announced the attack to those preparing to go on duty, and word-of-mouth traveled like a tidal wave, breaking the news that would stun and engulf everyone it touched.

It was Monday, 8 December, in the Philippines, but across the international date line on Hawaii, it was Sunday, 7 December 1941, the date that would live in infamy. At 0755 Hawaii time, naval and air forces of the empire of Japan attacked the military forces of the United States at Pearl Harbor and sank or damaged most of the U.S. Pacific Fleet. At the time of the Pearl Harbor attack, it was 0355 in the Philippines, and the islands were slowly awakening to the shock that America was at war and the Philippines would likely be Japan's next target.

Gen. Douglas MacArthur's adjutant had awakened Gen. Jonathan Wainwright with the news at 0435, and the military was awaiting MacArthur's orders. While the military commanders debated how to face the emergency, medical personnel went into action to prepare for the wounded they would care for when Japan turned its attention to the Philippines.

Lt. Josie Nesbit, acting chief nurse at the Sternberg General, was greeted by a group of upset nurses coming off the night shift. The women knew nurses and officers stationed at Pearl Harbor and were concerned that their friends might have been wounded or killed.

Nesbit was forty-seven-years old and had joined the Army Nurse Corps in 1918. She knew that her nurses would be badly needed in the coming hours. She told them, "Girls, you have to get to sleep today. You cannot stay here and weep and wail over this because you have to go to work tonight." She was glad to see the nurses settled down. "I don't know if they slept, but they quit crying anyhow."[1]

Only hours after their attack on Pearl Harbor, the Japanese struck at the Philippines, bombing Camp John Hay in the mountainous area of Baguio. That morning, the two army nurses stationed at the camp, Lts. Beatrice E. Chambers and Ruby G. Bradley, were getting ready for scheduled surgery and the day at the camp hospital. They were autoclaving the instruments at 0530 when Dr. Dana Wilson Nance was called to headquarters and informed that Pearl Harbor had been bombed. He returned to his office in the hospital and sent for Lieutenant Bradley. "Don't worry about your gown and gloves," he said. "I want to see you anyway, just keep them on." When Bradley arrived minutes later, he told her what had happened and added, "We could be hit any time here." Before the words were out of his mouth, the sound of approaching planes filled the air. Without thinking, the two ran to the door. "We could actually see the Japanese. We could recognize them as they were looking down at us because they were so close in those tiny planes," Lieutenant Bradley reported. The planes dropped more than fifty bombs, but luckily none hit the hospital itself. The dust they kicked up poured through the hospital's open windows and left one-quarter of an inch of fine powder on everything, making breathing in the hot, dusty air all but impossible for the next thirty minutes.[2]

The first casualty treated in the hospital was a one-year-old child. He and his mother were visiting on post when the first bombs fell and exploded a few feet from them. The little boy was in shock, and both his kneecaps were shattered. Dr. Nance worked on the unconscious child for some time with no response. "We'll have to rush through because we'll be getting other casualties," Dr. Nance said, and stepped away from the little boy.

"Do you think we could put some adrenalin in his heart?" Ruby Bradley asked.

"Yes, if you want to do it, go ahead and do it," Dr. Nance said.

Lieutenant Bradley got a syringe and looked at both the three-inch-long needle and the baby and decided she couldn't do it. At the same time she noticed a bottle of whiskey in the bottom of a medicine cabinet and the coffee pot and sugar on a stand next to it. A thought flashed through her mind, and she acted on it immediately. She put sugar on a piece of gauze, poured about a teaspoon of whiskey on it, and placed it in the baby's mouth. "He sucked it like everything, and it wasn't 5 minutes until he was as pink as a rose and yelling his head off." Above the baby's crying Lieutenant Bradley heard a wounded woman groaning and crying, "Where's my baby? Where's my baby?"

"Well, you hear him in there," Bradley answered. "He's all right now."[3]

About an hour later, news reached Sternberg and other army posts that Baguio had been bombed. By 0900, all nurses had been issued World War I helmets and gas masks. They were to wear the helmets and carry the gas masks, strapped around their waists, at all times.

Anxiety was high and only increased by having little to do while waiting. Some of the nurses decided to go on with their regular routine until they received orders to the contrary. At Fort McKinley Lts. Hattie Brantley and Minnie Breese were off duty until 1300. They had a reservation to play golf that morning, and neither could think of a reason to change their plans. "We'd have to wait for our generals and the Japs to decide what they'd do next," Lieutenant Brantley recalled. "So, we put our helmets and gas masks on and played golf. It probably helped the anxiety we felt, wondering what the Japs would do next, and the number of casualties that were sure to be the result."[4]

About 0700 Manila time, Colonel Brereton, commander of the

U.S. Air Forces in the Philippines, went to General MacArthur's headquarters at the edge of the old walled city and asked permission for his forces to conduct bombing raids on Japanese troop ships in Takao Harbor and on Japanese planes that were fogged in on Formosa. Brereton was told that no "offensive actions" could be authorized until MacArthur gave such orders, but he was permitted to order his B-17s and P-40 fighters into the air over the Philippine Islands to get them off the ground. One B-17 remained behind because it had generator problems. At 1100 Brereton received permission to arm his planes and carry out bombing missions. A coded message was sent to recall the planes, and they landed at Clark Field around 1145. Pilots and their crews went to lunch in the mess halls while maintenance workers refueled the planes and loaded bombs onto the B-17s. During this time the ailing B-17 had been repaired and took off to test the engine.

At approximately 1215, 192 Japanese warplanes, bombers, dive-bombers, and fighters flew over Clark Field, bombing and strafing the U.S. planes lined up in symmetrical patterns on the ground. Japanese pilots seemed to know exactly when and where the planes would be and bombed them into useless hulks. U.S. airpower in the Philippines was virtually destroyed on the ground nine hours after the attack on Pearl Harbor.

The only B-17 to survive the attack was the plane that had been grounded with generator trouble. It was on a test flight when Clark Field was attacked and was hidden on another Philippine airfield in hope it could be used later against the Japanese.

The first wave of the attack lasted fourteen minutes and left 85 dead and 350 wounded. Stotsenberg had only three or four ambulances, but corpsmen and troops used trucks and cars to bring the wounded to the hospital. The nurses not already on duty rushed to the hospital, despite a second wave of Japanese planes that attacked Clark Field three minutes after the first raid had ended.

When word of the bombing at Clark Field reached the Sternberg, nurses were called into the assembly hall and volunteers were requested to go to Stotsenberg to help care for the wounded. Two nurses, 2d Lts. Phyllis Arnold and Helen Cassiani, the latter a twenty-four-year-old from Bridgewater, Massachusetts, were sent as a surgical team; Arnold was an anesthetist and Cassiani a surgical nurse. Lt. Anna Williams was detailed as a general duty nurse.

The group, which included four physicians and several corpsmen, rode along the back roads in a school bus to a town just outside Clark Field. They traveled on secondary roads because they would offer more cover should the Japanese planes return to the area. Filipinos lined the road in the small town of Wimevaro and flashed victory signs at the party.

By this time, it was dark and the bus used its lights only when absolutely necessary. They crossed the airfield by moonlight. Everyone on the bus was getting very tense so they began to sing old World War I songs. "When we got to the airfield, there were our B-17s . . . burnt. They looked like dinosaur skeletons," Phyllis Arnold recalled. "We found the hospital by the moans and the cries of the wounded." The operating room was in a large tent and under blackout conditions. The surgical teams had been on duty for about nine hours so the new arrivals took over immediately. Within minutes, Lieutenant Arnold had her first taste of the realities of war. "My first case was a spinal. . . . It was a young sergeant who had been on another [air] field and his feet were strafed. . . . He asked me if this would take him out of the war. I couldn't answer him because I knew he was going to lose his feet. That was when I began to realize we were at war—look at this—this young man. We worked all night."[5]

Nurses and physicians worked around the clock caring for the wounded. Officers and men were heartsick that so many had been killed and wounded because the planes had been "sitting ducks" for the enemy. Japanese "sleepers," planted months and even years before, had aided the Japanese by providing accurate intelligence concerning the military sites in the Philippines. Lt. Anna Williams recalled how upset the commander of the air corps was after the terrible attack.

"I do remember very vividly that I had met the officer . . . a colonel, who was in charge of the Air Corps there at the Clark Field.

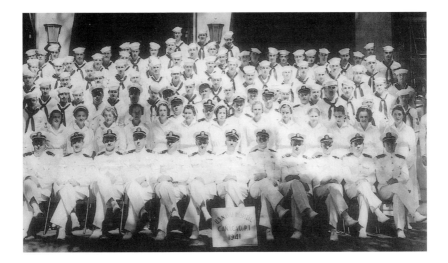

U.S. Naval Hospital staff at Canacao, P.I., 1941. Navy nurses in second row, from left to right: Todd, Bernatitis, Taylor, Yarnell, Ordman, Cobb, Still, O'Haver, Harrington, Metcalf, Chapman, Dwyer; U.S. Navy photograph.

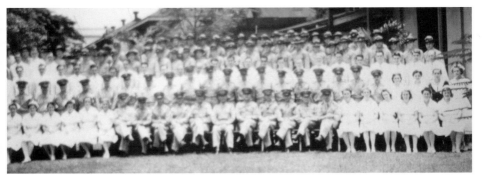

Pre-World War II Army Medical Personnel, Philippine Island Command; U.S. Army Signal Corps.

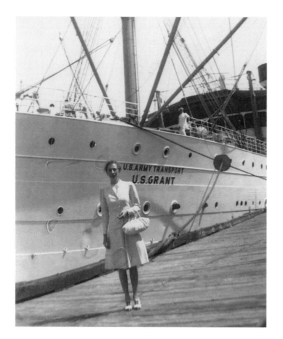

2d Lt. Frances Nash ready to board the USS *Grant* for her trip to the Philippine Islands; authors' archives.

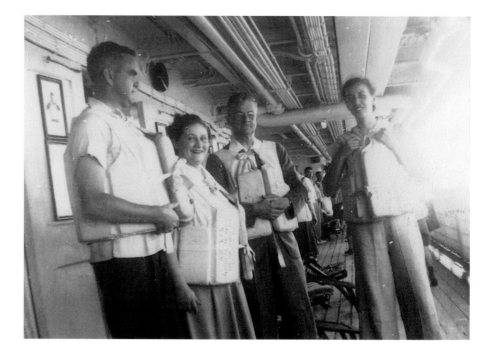

2d Lt. Frances Nash (far right) and her military traveling companions aboard the USS *Grant* during a lifeboat drill; authors' archives.

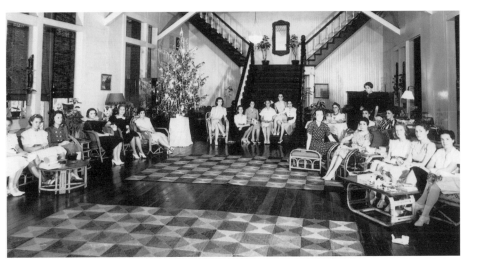

Army nurses in nurses' quarters living room at Sternberg General Hospital, Manila, Philippine Islands, 1939; Armed Forces Institute of Pathology.

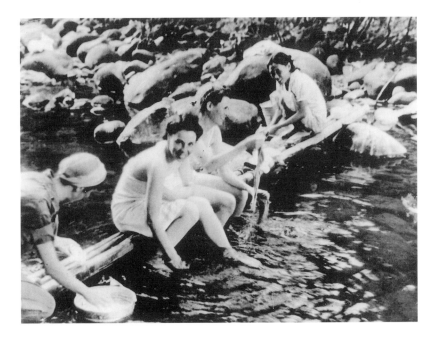

Nurses on Bataan bathing and doing their laundry in a jungle stream; World Wide.

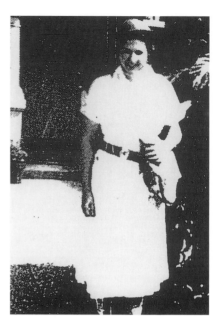

2d Lt. Hattie R. Brantley, Manila, December 1941, wearing a World War I helmet, with gas mask at her side; authors' archives.

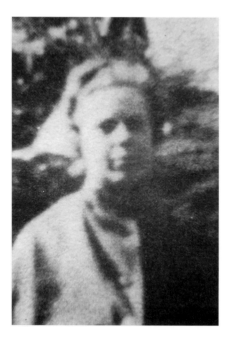

2d Lt. Madeline Ullom, Corregidor, Philippine Islands, 1941; authors' archives.

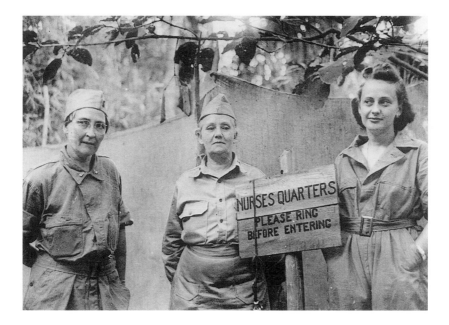

1st Lt. Josephine Nesbit, Capt. Maude C. Davison, and 2d Lt. Helen Hennessey at Hospital No.2 on Bataan, January 1942; International News Photo.

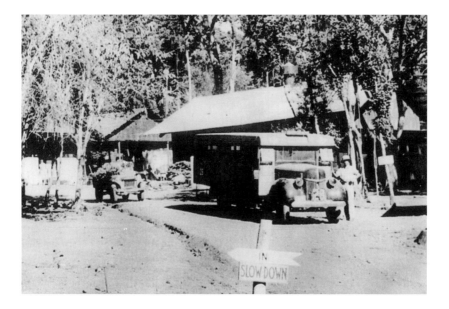

Field Hospital No.2 on Bataan, 1942; U.S. Army Signal Corps.

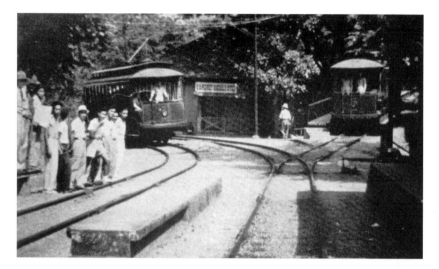

Pre-war Corregidor with trolleys that ran between Bottomside and Topside; National Archives.

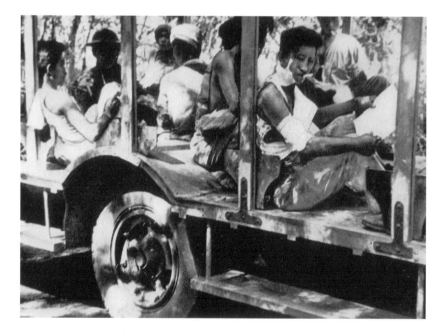

Philippine buses were used to transport wounded soldiers on Bataan; U.S. Army Signal Corps.

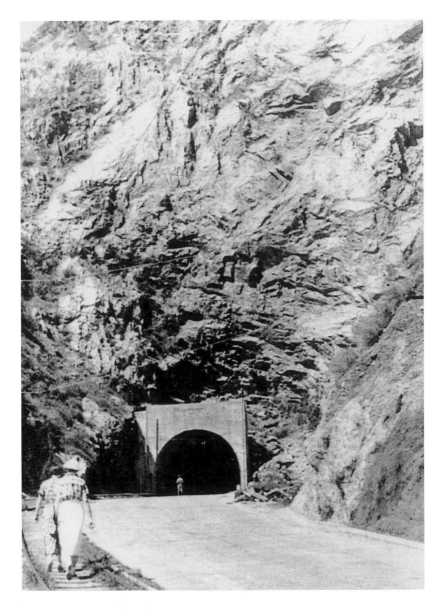

One of the entrances to Malinta Tunnel showing the rock of Corregidor that served as part of the tunnel's protection from Japanese bombs and artillery shells; U.S. Army Signal Corps.

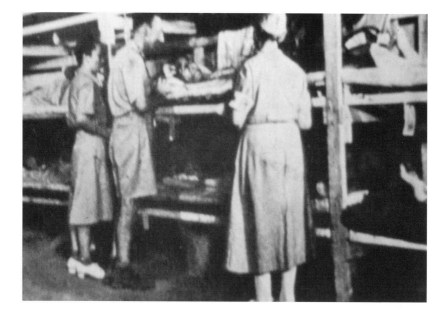

Army nurses and doctor caring for wounded troops in Malinta Tunnel, Corregidor; U.S. Army Signal Corps.

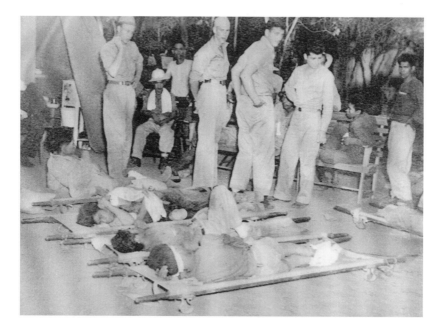

Wounded Filipino soldiers on Bataan awaiting medical attention; U.S. Army Signal Corps.

[This was most likely Brereton.] I can recall how really down he was because he had wanted to get his men up in the planes. They knew that the Japanese were coming and he wanted to get his men up off the ground, and he wasn't allowed to because war hadn't been declared. He was really desolate. . . . They [the men] said MacArthur wouldn't allow him to take the planes up. Consequently, his men were caught on the ground, and many of them were killed or injured. I don't know statistics on this but I just know that we had lots of injured men, and he was very, very dejected."[6]

Rumors passed quickly at Stotsenberg that the Japanese were going to stage a landing at Clark Field. Nurses could not spend time worrying because they were too busy taking care of the casualties. It became increasingly obvious that white duty uniforms were not made for treating the wounded under combat conditions. Several of the nurses told a male officer that they needed clothes to replace the nurses' white uniforms. The officer offered air corps coveralls, and the nurses went to the warehouse to collect them. Since all the coveralls were large sizes, the nurses used their off duty time to take them in at the belt.[7] The same day, nurses were issued combat boots and dog tags for the first time. A day later, they were moving patients who could be transported aboard trains that would deliver them to Sternberg General Hospital in Manila.

At Canacao Navy Hospital on Cavite, Lt. Bertha Evans received a phone call at 0600 from her boyfriend, a line officer at Cavite Navy Yard, ten miles across the bay from Manila. He told her "Bertha, Pearl Harbor has been bombed. We've been up all night with the admiral." Evans, who had to be on duty at 0630, awakened as many nurses as she could with the news, "We're at war with Japan."[8]

At 0730 the eleven navy nurses at Cavite gathered to hear the news officially. They were issued helmets and gas masks along with pamphlets telling how to detect poisonous gasses and care for gassed patients. A decontamination chamber was set up in a general ward and drills were conducted on how to respond in case of a mustard gas attack.

White duty uniforms were replaced with dungarees and blue work shirts, but according to Lt. Edwina Todd, not every nurse appreciated the exchange. "Peggy [Nash] said she'd die before she'd wear those." That resolve did not last long. As the war progressed, the wisdom of this new "uniform" became more evident. Lt. Evans recalled the first Japanese bombs that fell within hearing distance of the hospital at Cavite: "When they came over and bombed Clark Field, that's the first time we heard the bombs. We were downstairs. They had cots for us. And we were wearing our dungarees. We had our helmets and our flashlights down beside our bunks. When we heard those bombs at Clark Field, we all rolled off the bed we were so excited. I remember I couldn't find my shoes, I couldn't find my helmet, couldn't find my flashlight for several minutes. . . ."[9]

Fifteen hundred miles away, only fifteen minutes after the first bombs fell on Pearl Harbor, approximately nine Japanese planes dropped bombs on Guam, where the garrison of five hundred marines and sailors had no artillery. The bombing and strafing continued for two days. The Navy Department received the last message from Guam on 9 December 1941 at 1530 (island time): "Last attack centered at Agana. Civilians machine-gunned in streets. Two native wards of hospital and hospital compound machine-gunned. Building in which Japanese nationals are confined bombed."[10]

The attack sent large numbers of wounded sailors, marines, and civilians to the hospital. The five navy nurses who were assigned to the hospital cared for scores of wounded within the first hour.

Around 1000 on 10 December, five thousand Japanese troops landed, and street-to-street combat began in the capital city of Agana, where the naval hospital was located. When the firing ceased around dawn the next day, the navy nurses were among the horrified witnesses who saw the Japanese flag raised in front of the hospital compound. The nurses were advised to remove the gold braid from their caps to prevent the Japanese from knowing they were military personnel. The action was hardly necessary because it never occurred to the Japanese that women could be military officers.

The Japanese set up their headquarters inside the hospital, reasoning that should the Americans counterattack, they would not bomb the naval hospital. The conquerors took over all hospital wards, leaving only one for use by natives and Americans. The navy nurses were permitted to care for the patients and to remain in their living quarters when not on duty. Japanese naval officers, sailors, and soldiers made frequent unannounced inspections at all hours of the day and night.

Japanese troops were allowed to run uncontrolled looting the city. When nothing of value remained to be stolen, Japanese officers made a show of calling a halt to the looting and were frequently observed slapping their enlisted personnel. This disregard for the dignity of their own troops was replicated in the treatment of their captives. Because the Imperial Army's senior officers disrespected and mistreated junior officers, who in turn mistreated those lower in rank, it was inevitable that Japanese captives would be treated with disrespect and brutality.

Like all Japanese prisoners of war, nurses were compelled to bow from the waist when meeting or passing Japanese officers and guards. Anyone who did not obey was punished on the spot. Lt. Virginia J. Forgerty was slapped by a Japanese sailor when she failed to understand an order.[11]

A few days after the occupation began, the chief nurse, Marian Olds, a graduate of George Washington University, who had fifteen years of experience in the navy, was told to have her four nurses assemble in the plaza with the native Chamorro nurses. The navy nurses readied themselves for the worst. They had seen men stripped, searched, and bayoneted by Japanese soldiers; they had watched women bayoneted when they had not gotten out of the way of the Japanese quickly enough; and they had no reason to believe they would be treated differently.

Despite the atrocities, Navy Nurse Corps officers maintained a calm demeanor and helped the wounded as best they could. Lt. Leona Jackson expressed the feelings of all the nurses when she said, "This was the time for which we had trained all of these years, the Final

Examination in the School of Professional Experience. It was a strange sensation to look upon yourself reacting automatically to situations, keeping a quiet voice in the midst of consternation." [12]

Considering what might have been their plight, the nurses were slightly relieved when they were taken to the Officers' Club, located on a hill, and given demonstrations of machine-gun fire and flame-throwing. They were not impressed.

Back at Canacao, navy nurses faced their first enemy air attack. At 1200 on 10 December, the air raid siren sounded as fifty-four Japanese bombers and fighters attacked Cavite Navy Yard. Lt. Edwina Todd remembered the onslaught: "They looked beautiful against the blue sky until we realized that we were the target." [13]

Sandbags had been placed around the open area beneath the nurses' quarters, and as the planes dropped their bombs on the navy yard, nurses who were in their quarters or having lunch ran to take cover under the building. As they listened to the sound of exploding bombs, the women feared that if the Japanese hit the ammunition depot at Cavite, the concussion from the explosion would kill them.

When bombs fell on Sangley Point and the radio station between the yard and the navy hospital, the ground under the nurses' quarters shook. Luckily, none of the bombs hit the hospital, but the navy yard was leveled, and casualties were high. The raid was conducted in several waves and lasted almost an hour.

When the nurses ran to the hospital after the raid, they were surprised at how many casualties had already been brought in for treatment. Dorothy Still, a twenty-seven-year-old nurse from Long Beach, California remembered: "The wards were overflowing with patients. They were lying on boards, old doors, corrugated roofing materials, or just anything a patient could be moved on. We had Filipino [Filipina] women and children in addition to Navy personnel injured in the Yard out on the Point. . . ." [14]

Nurses were ordered to administer one-quarter grain of morphine to all patients and to place those needing surgery in the hallways because there was no space for them elsewhere. Medical personnel worked around the clock caring for the wounded, who arrived in a seemingly endless stream. Nurses were pressed into giving care and making decisions customarily restricted to physicians, but unlike physicians, nurses before Pearl Harbor did not carry stethoscopes. This lack made some decisions hard because life-and-death judgments had to be made minute by minute. Lieutenant Evans recalled that in one case she could not find a pulse on a wounded man. After asking Lt. Margaret Nash to check for a pulse and being told she could not find one either, they called a corpsman to take the body to the morgue. Halfway there the wounded sailor sat up on the stretcher and asked an astonished medic, "Where am I?" The sailor recovered from his wounds, but Evans and Nash never forgot the incident. "If we had a stethoscope," Evans said, "we could have heard the heart."[15]

When daylight ran out, medical personnel worked by flashlight and battle lantern until the hospital's commanding officer, Capt. Robert Davis, ordered that all lights be turned on so the staff could work faster at evacuating Canacao's patients. Days later the nurses learned from Davis that the Japanese had delivered an ultimatum to Canacao: the hospital must be evacuated within thirty-six hours or it would be declared a military objective. After all sick and wounded had been transferred to Estado Mayor, an army base adjacent to Sternberg General, the navy nurses left Cavite by boat and set up a temporary hospital at the Philippine Union College in Balintawac, a suburb of Manila.[16]

As time went on, all regular military hospitals except the Sternberg were closed and their patients and nurses were sent to the Sternberg or one of eight annexes that were created as emergency receiving stations. The annexes were designated by letters A through H and located as follows: A—Jai Alai Center, 250 beds; B—Estada Mayor, 600 beds; C—Girls' Dormitory, 400 beds; D—Philippine Women's University, 500 beds; E—Santa Scholastica, 450 beds; F—Fort William McKinley, 250 beds; G—Holy Ghost, 400 beds; H—LaSallee Extension University, 575 beds. Each annex was assigned specific types of patients, although the lines often blurred. Minor casualties went to one annex, medical patients to another, navy casualties to Santa Scholastica and so on. Two annexes were staffed but never received patients because General MacArthur called for the evacuation of Manila before they were needed.[17]

The operating rooms at the Sternberg stayed busy around the clock with nurses working eighteen to twenty hours a day. Lt. Madeline Ullom recalled, "I often slept on the operating table, or just put a pad in a corner and slept while things were quiet." Someone finally pointed out that there was no end in sight for casualties, and nurses were allowed to return to their quarters for an hour or two of sleep during the infrequent lulls in surgery.[18]

On 12 December the Japanese made their first landing in the Philippines at Aparri, on the northern tip of Luzon, and on the following day, they attacked the beaches at Vigan, north of Lingayen Gulf, and began landing troops and supplies from eighty-four transports. The B-17 that had escaped destruction at Clark Field attacked the Japanese landing but was doomed to failure because it was the lone American plane against the entire Nipponese attack force.

The personnel of Camp John Hay at Baguio were notified that they probably would have to evacuate in a few days because the Japanese navy was headed for Lingayen Gulf. "We could see the ships coming in [to] the Lingayen Gulf. There . . . [were] 84 of them there," Lt. Ruby Bradley said. Bradley was thirty-four years old and had been an army nurse for seven years. "You could go out to the road and look down and see them. . . . Everyday they'd say, 'Well, they're coming up the mountain.' Everyday they would shell the gulf a little bit there to delay their coming. We weren't too sure that they weren't outside the city when we left that morning. We were supplied and the day before we left, they fitted the two of us [nurses] with combat boots."[19]

Before leaving for the mountains to join the guerrillas who sympathized with the Americans against the Japanese, the nurses and Dr. Nance sent as much medical equipment as possible, surgical instruments and supplies, even the x-ray machine, to Notre Dame Hospital, Baguio's civilian facility. Approximately fifty people were in the group that evacuated the hospital. During the first leg of the

journey, the party traveled in several vehicles, but as they continued their ascent on the winding and narrowing mountain road,
the refugees were forced to abandon and destroy their conveyances.

They walked on a path just wide enough to allow them to place
one foot in front of the other. As Bradley negotiated this hazard-
ous trail with its frequent precipices, she asked one of the sergeants,
"What'd happen if our foot would slip?" The sergeant was quick to
respond, "It depended on your past life, because it was no hope
there [of surviving]." Falling to one's death was not the only danger along the trail. "Once when we had to cross a little river, we had
to cross many," Ruby Bradley recalled, "there were Japanese planes
going over us. We dispersed a little bit into the bushes every time
we'd hear one coming."[20]

The refugees had been deprived of sleep since the war had begun two weeks earlier, and they soon became tired from walking.
At one point during their climb, they were overtaken by two U.S.
Army engineers whom they had known at Camp John Hay. These
two men were hiking at a fast pace and soon disappeared far ahead
of them. Three hours later, the group saw a donkey coming down
the trail. "It had a sign on it," Bradley said. "'For the nurses.' The
little donkey was so small that if one of us got on it, we'd break his
back." The nurses decided to use the donkey to carry a soldier whose
feet were so badly blistered that he refused to walk any farther. "He
was so tall and his legs were so long, that we had to tie them up,
and tie him on," Ruby Bradley explained. "Beatrice [Chambers]
got in front of the donkey, and I got in back of it, and we tried to
get the donkey to move." They finally succeeded and walked on for
an hour or two before stopping for a rest.[21]

Dr. Nance, Bradley, and four or five others went on ahead to a
lumber camp where a Filipino family had lived and worked for
years. The family allowed several of the party to stay in their home.
"They had a little house where we slept on the kitchen floor," Bradley said, "which is sort of peculiar because here were two young
men, perhaps American-Filipinos, who had two of the finest beds
in the whole place. The next night, they gave us the beds. Then the
following night, the commanding officer came across there and he

was really in bad shape, so we put him in the bed, and we slept on the floor."[22]

American troops passed through the lumber camp in the next couple of days, and the two nurses treated their blistered feet and contemplated their own future.

On 22 December the Japanese began landing their main forces at Lingayen Gulf, 130 miles northeast of Manila. Japanese bombing raids over Manila and along the waterfront intensified. Army and navy nurses saw more and more wounded brought to them for care, and fires raged throughout the city.

3

Descent into Hell

We were in the situation and it doesn't do any good to wring your hands and say how terrible it is and "What's going on?" and "Why don't they do something?" and "Isn't it awful!" You just roll up your sleeves and do what you can to make better the situation that you're in.

Lt. Col. Madeline Ullom, USA, NC (Ret.)

On 23 December at approximately 1800, General MacArthur left Manila and moved his headquarters to the rock fortress of Corregidor, at the mouth of Manila Bay. Less than an hour before, MacArthur had decided that to prevent the destruction of Manila, he would declare it an "open city." A member of MacArthur's staff telephoned Gen. Jonathan Wainwright and told him that War Plan Orange 3 was in effect. American and Filipino forces would make the desperate retreat to Bataan, planned more than a decade earlier.

Army and navy nurses were among the last to learn the news. Lt. Hattie Brantley recalled the moment her group was informed: "During the evening meal of December 23, our hospital C.O. said, 'Girls, pack your white duty uniforms in a duffel bag because we're going to Bataan tomorrow.' Most of us had never even heard of Bataan. So, on the morning of Christmas Eve, we loaded into buses and open trucks, dressed in our white duty uniforms, a World War I helmet on our heads, and a gas mask at our sides, and headed for the Bataan Peninsula."[1]

Not all the military nurses left for Bataan, and not all those who did, traveled the same way or took the same route. Several army nurses were left in Manila to help equip a ship that would carry wounded patients to Australia. Before the ship, the *Mactan*, departed Manila, they were issued identification cards stating that they were detailed to help with the Red Cross ship. The ship was an old minesweeper with an engine that showed its age. The Army Medical Department had radioed Tokyo and asked permission for a merchant ship loaded with wounded to sail to Australia around the end of the month. Though the request was not answered, they decided to undertake the trip anyway.

Col. Percey J. Carroll, M.D., supervised the acquisition and loading of the *Mactan*. He requested that Lt. Florence MacDonald furnish him with an army nurse who was skilled at improvising. She would be the only army nurse on board if and when the *Mactan* sailed for Darwin.

While other nurses set off for Bataan on the morning of 24 December, Lt. Frances L. Nash, a tall, dark-haired, thirty-year-old army nurse from Wilkes County, Georgia, was called by her commanding officer, Col. J.W. Duckworth, and given special instructions. "It was Christmas Eve when I was told to prepare myself to be taken prisoner. Five years before, I would have laughed at the thought of ever receiving such an order, and answering merely, 'Yes, Sir.' My commanding officer . . . told me I was to remain until all staff members and supplies had been evacuated. 'In case you are cut off, you must prepare to be taken prisoner,' he said."[2]

All day on Christmas Eve and Christmas Day, Lieutenant Nash worked in surgery and in her spare time destroyed any papers that might prove useful to the Japanese. On Christmas night, the enemy was drawing closer to Manila and the number of wounded increasing, but Nash and the rest of the staff were ordered to leave Manila and join Hospital No. 2 on Bataan. They climbed aboard a small inner-island steamer at 2300 and began their zigzagging trip across Manila Bay. The red and yellow glow from burning buildings on shore and flaming ships in the bay added to the light cast on the water by a brightly shining moon. Nash had vivid memories of that trip.

> What sleep I got that night, I caught stretched out on the top deck, clad in mechanic's overalls, helmet and gas mask, my pockets full of medicine, stimulants, narcotics and a tourniquet in case of an accident during the crossing. For a moment, as I lay there looking up at the stars, I couldn't visualize the fact that everything wasn't peaceful; yet all I had to do was turn my head to the side to know it was not.
>
> During the night we passed Corregidor and saw fires burning on the topside. At 10 A.M. the next morning, we arrived at Bataan's Lamao docks under a blanket of Jap bombers, with fighters strafing our little boat. As we hit the docks, we all dove for cover. I already had been in ditches and under bridges at Fort McKinley, but all I could see on the docks was a sort of native scoop under which chickens had taken refuge. Without thinking twice, I pushed the chickens out, feathers flying, and squeezed in myself. It's funny to think of now; it wasn't funny then.[3]

Lt. Frances L. Nash carried enough morphine with her to provide each army nurse with a lethal dose, which each wore hidden in her hair from that point until their liberation from Santo Tomas Internment Camp in February 1945. The morphine was the nurses' edge against an enemy they all knew only too well could be brutal in the manner it dealt death to its captives. As long as the nurses could remain useful to their patients and maintain their dignity, the morphine would remain their secret.

Since most army nurses had left for Bataan, Captain Davis ordered all navy nurses to report to Santa Scholastica College, where the army had set up a hospital. With the exception of Ann Bernatitis, a member of the only navy medical team assigned to Bataan, navy nurses were to care for the critical and bed patients left behind when the army evacuated the city. The patients to leave on the *Mactan* would be selected from this group.

For those army and navy nurses who remained in Manila after the military pulled out, each day was filled with the stress of knowing that Japanese troops would enter the city in a matter of days, if not hours. While navy nurses cared for the wounded at Santa Scholastica, army nurses worked as fast as possible getting the *Mactan* ready to carry several hundred wounded to safety.

Meanwhile, hidden in the mountains near Baguio, Lts. Ruby Bradley and Beatrice Chambers and their host family were sent a Christmas dinner, including turkey, by a second lumber camp family. The nurses asked the family for permission to share their own portions with the eight American soldiers staying on the grounds outside.

The evacuees' original plan was to join the guerrillas by hiking higher into the mountains via Balady Pass. This strategy was derailed when the Japanese army tanks engaged and obliterated the Filipino horse cavalry at Balady Pass. Now that the enemy held the pass, the group was cut off from the guerrillas.

A day after Christmas, news of increasing numbers of casualties in Baguio reached the mountain lumber camp. It was decided that the nurses and several military personnel would return to Camp John Hay to give medical attention to the women and children in the area. When the group completed the winding descent and reached the foot of the mountain, they were met by Japanese troops and a line of their army trucks. The American men were loaded onto the trucks, the nurses placed in an officer's sedan, and all were taken to Brent School in Baguio.

Foreseeing difficult conditions at the hands of the Japanese, Lt. Beatrice Chambers had taken it upon herself to procure some food. "I found a big ham in Brent School's kitchen. I went down there and I stole that ham and put it under my shirt and acted as if I was pregnant and walked out with that ham. . . . We had no uniforms. I had an old army shirt on and army pants on, cavalry pants. . . . [We looked] just like missionaries."[4]

Those at Brent School had a close brush with death when the Japanese, who had already isolated the men in one group, separated the women from the children. Chambers remembered those harrowing moments: "They had the machine guns on us, and they were going to get [kill] us all. . . . Fortunately, a Jap major came along and decided he was going to make us hostages."[5]

On 29 December, carrying their meager baggage, the captives started their march toward their first internment camp. The Japanese had trucks and automobiles in the area but chose to humiliate their five hundred prisoners by forcing them to march. Men, women, children, and American military personnel walked the approximately two miles to Scout Hill at Camp John Hay, where they would be interned for several months.

The camp had sustained bombing damage, but four separate barracks remained standing. Each barracks was constructed to house fifty men. The Japanese crowded all five hundred prisoners into one barracks while the other three remained empty. There were no lights, no sanitary facilities, no water, and no food.

Through the kindness of several Japanese civilians in the area, a truck was sent from Baguio carrying canned foods and water, and the prisoners had a meal. That night they made themselves as comfortable as possible given the lack of beds and blankets. Since Baguio and Camp John Hay lay at an altitude of five thousand feet, nights were cold, and internees suffered considerably before they were able to obtain adequate bed coverings.[6]

In the hot, humid weather of southern Luzon and Corregidor the battle was still raging. On 29 December the Japanese bombed Corregidor for the first time, dropping sixty thousand tons of bombs on the Topside installation, including a few that fell near and on the hospital. The move of the hospital to the relative safety of Malinta Tunnel was quickly completed.

In the early morning hours of 30 December, all but one of the army nurses remaining in Manila were evacuated to Corregidor. Lt. Madeline Ullom spoke vividly of that evacuation:

It was about 2 A.M. when we were awakened and told to pack whatever we could into our musette bags and go downstairs to the front door. We were not to turn any lights on. So, I think there were ten of us; we gathered downstairs and waited. We could hear tanks rolling by outside, and I wanted to look at them. I went to the porch door and looked out. They were our tanks, and they were retreating through Manila.

They took us down to the waterfront in an ambulance. The only light was moonlight, as the driver tried to avoid bomb craters. We finally reached the dock where the *Don Estaban*, a small inner island boat, was waiting to take us to Corregidor.

It wasn't an easy trip because the Japanese were strafing the waterfront and the bay. Some of our ships had been sunk in the harbor and the captain of the boat dodged around the torn and battered hulks. I'm sure all of us were hoping the hulls of the large ships would hide us from the Japanese planes that were bombing and strafing all around us.

Just as the sky began to turn gray, the captain told us we were going through the minefield. As soon as we docked, an air raid siren went off and believe me, we got off that boat pretty quickly. In just a minute or two a truck came by and without actually stopping—they just slowed down—they grabbed us, lifted us onto the truck and took us to Malinta Tunnel.[7]

Lt. Josephine Nesbit, a native of Butler, Missouri, discovered that the evacuation to Corregidor endangered more than lives. As anyone who has ever spent time in the military knows, one's pay and health records are of vital importance. When the Don Estaban arrived at the Corregidor docks, Nesbit was not among the nurses picked up and carried to Malinta Tunnel by army trucks. "When we disembarked from the boat at North Dock on Corregidor, the air raid alert sounded," she said. "I was carrying all of the nurses' records in a large cardboard box. A colonel jumped out of his jeep and told me to drop the box, and take cover during the alert. I started to protest, 'But. . . .' He grabbed the box, threw it to the ground, grabbed my arm, loaded me into his jeep and drove to the Navy Tunnel." When the all clear sounded, the colonel drove Nesbit back to North Dock and left to take care of more pressing duties. "I heaved a sigh of relief and thanked God that the box containing all the nurses' records was still there. I picked it up and someone gave me a lift to Malinta Tunnel Hospital."[8]

In Manila on 31 December the army patients at Santa Scholastica were evacuated to the *Mactan.* The ship was loaded with 375 seriously wounded, one army nurse, Lt. Floramund Fellmuth, eight Filipino doctors, eight Filipina nurses, and Colonel Carroll. Lt. Edwina Todd spoke of that time with sadness: "The last of these patients left the hospital at 2030; it was hard to see so many amputees and paralyzed men left behind, only to become prisoner of the Japanese."[9]

Corregidor was notified that the *Mactan* was sailing out of Manila Bay to Australia. Unfortunately, one of Corregidor's artillery batteries did not get the message and was preparing to shell the ship. The battery finally got the word, and the *Mactan* sailed unscathed out of Manila Bay.

Less than two hours after the ship was at sea, the wounded began calling for doctors and nurses and complaining that they were in great pain. The medical staff began removing dressings and discovered that the patients were infested with ants. The entire ship was crawling with ants. Despite the scarcity of medical supplies, all bandages had to be changed immediately and the ship treated to rid it of the six-legged pests.

Once the ship had passed Celebes, its aged engine became overheated. Great billows of black smoke came from belowdecks. Luckily, there was a Filipino doctor on board who had studied engineering before medicine, and he managed to repair the engine.

The next catastrophe was a storm that struck the ship in the Macassar Straits and almost sank her. In addition, there was the ever-present danger that a Japanese torpedo would sink her before she reached Australia. The chosen port of debarkation was Darwin, but when it was learned that Darwin was under Japanese attack, the route was altered. Despite all the adverse forces, the *Mactan* miraculously disembarked her passengers safely in Sydney weeks after leaving Manila.[10]

Time and the enemy were not so kind to the patients and navy medical personnel left behind in Manila. On New Year's Eve the American flag flying over Santa Scholastica was hauled down and burned to prevent its falling into Japanese hands. Japanese troops entered Manila on 1 January 1942. Lt. Edwina Todd remembered that day: "New Year's Day ushered in a new life for us. Across the street where Japanese prisoners had been quartered we saw them released; they all shouted 'Banzai' and waved miniature Rising Sun Flags at us as the Japanese Army marched in."[11]

On the second of January Japanese troops entered Santa Scholastica. "The next day we were prisoners," Todd said. "Our men were immediately set to work stringing barbed wire to fence us in. At night Jap sentries moved through our sleeping quarters every half-hour stamping their feet as they walked to insure that you didn't sleep. Sometimes you would awaken to find a bayonet stuck through your mosquito netting and a Jap sentry leering over you."[12]

One of the horrors the navy nurses witnessed in their first days of captivity was the attitude of the Japanese toward seriously wounded and helpless patients. "When we refused to let them kill the wounded," Todd said, "they asked us to kill them." Patients were frequently struck if they did not rise out of their bunks at the command of Japanese soldiers. One soldier might shadow-box with the patients, while another soldier, with fixed bayonet, stood by in case a wounded American or Filipino should be so foolish as to strike back.[13]

The navy nurses were ordered to take inventory of all medical supplies. Two days later the Japanese checked the stores against that list. What the Japanese did not know, and fortunately did not find out, was that the nurses had listed only about 75 percent of the most important medicines, such as quinine. "We covered this loss by breaking one of the cardinal rules of pharmacy," Edwina Todd said, "mislabeling drugs. Most of our quinine was labeled soda bicarbonate." During their captivity at Santa Scholastica, four Filipino patients escaped. The Japanese quickly posted notices stating that for every patient who escaped in the future, the patient on each side of his bed and the nurse on the ward would be shot. There were no more escapes.[14]

4

The Other Alamo

Those nurses of Bataan and Corregidor, what can possibly be said worthy of them?
Col. Carlos P. Romulo, aide-de-camp to General MacArthur

One late afternoon during the hottest December in the history of Bataan, twelve Pambusco buses discharged their passengers and the nurses and medical personnel got their first look at the Limay beach area. The compound consisted of twenty one-story wooden barracks with palm-thatched roofs and open, glass-free windows with lightweight palm closings that could be raised or lowered like shades. One corrugated tin warehouse stood in contrast to the long, narrow, framed barracks. These buildings, deserted and virtually empty, had once served as Camp Limay, a training facility for Filipino Scouts.

The nurses claimed one of these barracks for their quarters. It was divided into small rooms with four or five beds scattered through them. "Oh, no!" one of the twenty-five nurses said in an exhausted voice. "Does this mean we sleep on the floor?" One of the medics whose bus had arrived earlier at the compound motioned toward the warehouse. "There are beds and linen in there."

An army truck pulled up in front of the nurses' barracks and stopped. "The Quartermaster thought you might be able to use these," a young corporal said as he dropped two large boxes inside the door. The nurses set upon the cartons like bees on honeysuckle. Lieutenant Brantley led the swarm.

"Army Air Corps coveralls. All size forty-two," she said. "Remember the belts were stretched across the back from side to side. And the front is best described by the modern day adage of 'hang loose'! Letha McHale got lost and wasn't seen for quite a while when she tried on a pair. On Rosemary Hogan, they looked tailor-made, a perfect fit. And the rest of us were somewhere in between. We hung loose!"[1]

Attired in their new army field uniforms, the nurses headed for the warehouse where the medic had indicated they would find cots and bedding. It was there, but headboards, footboards, and joining bars were piled in separate stacks, and it took many trips between the warehouse and the barracks before each nurse had an assembled cot to sleep on that night.

After a quick supper of field pancakes, the nurses gathered on the beach and looked across Manila Bay. The sky was bright with fingers of fire reaching high into the night. The military at the Cavite Naval Base were exploding ammunition dumps and setting fire to fuel so they would not fall into enemy hands. The nurses wondered what was happening at the Army-Navy Club, the Manila Hotel, and other familiar spots. "We also wondered what was happening to us," Hattie Brantley said. She spoke in a pleasant East Texas accent. "But let me say quickly that the main theme then, there and forever after was 'Help is on the way!' We evidenced faith, hope, and trust in God, in General MacArthur, in F.D.R. and in the U.S.A. In fact, anytime anyone looked in the direction of the bay and did not see a convoy steaming in, it was with disbelief! And with the certainty that this convoy would arrive at least by tomorrow."[2]

At sunup on Christmas Day, the nurses, doctors, medics, and all available hands went into the warehouse and dug out the gear for the hospital. They were shocked to discover how old the equipment that was to serve the casualties of a new war appeared. "There were old iron cots, rusty and dirty, and I'll swear they were packed in 1918 newspapers," Hattie Brantley said.

Only later did nurses and medical personnel learn about War Plan Orange 3. "This War Plan Orange-3 which we knew nothing about other than the fact that it was now activated, had been talked about and planned in all departments except the medical department," Brantley said. "There were surgical instruments packed in Cosmolene. They wasted an awful lot of good ether, cleaning those instruments, getting the Cosmolene off so that they could be used in surgery."[3]

Bataan was fast becoming a site of preparations and action. On 26 December 1941, Colonel Duckworth, known affectionately as "the Duck," sent a request to 2d Lt. Frances L. Nash to report to him at Hospital No.1. Nash was on her way to join nineteen other nurses and a medical team to set up Field Hospital No.2 in the jungle south of Limay. Duckworth requested that she report instead to Hospital No.1 to supervise the organization and operation of the surgical units. Nash, a veteran of the emergency rooms at Grady Memorial Hospital in Atlanta, reported for duty at Hospital No. 1 that same day.

The nurses and medical teams set up eighteen of the barracks with thirty to forty cots each, and by 28 December 1941, each ward was filled to overflowing with front-line casualties. The surgery, which was equipped for blackout conditions, worked around the clock.

General Wainwright's divisions had been fighting north of Bataan but were unable to hold the line against the Japanese. The Allied forces retreated to Bataan early on the morning of 6 January, and the medical and surgical supplies stopped arriving from Manila. The Japanese had cut the supply lines as they drove southward. The one thing that continued to be delivered to the hospital in ever-increasing numbers was the wounded.

By the second week in January, wards were no longer designated "medical" or "surgical"; every ward had surgical patients. One nurse and two medics were assigned to each ward, and the ratio between medical staff and casualties grew larger every day. The regular work shift rose from twelve to twenty hours in length. To accommodate the increasing flow of casualties, patients were moved five miles south to Hospital No.2 by ambulance, truck, or bus as soon as they were in condition to be transported. Cots were filled as quickly as they were vacated. Beds literally had no time to cool off between patients.

Lt. Bertha Dworsky, a thirty-year-old native of Hallettsville, Texas, remarked on one aspect of that stressful situation: "We were just a big happy family there. Each time they would bring in casualties, they were usually people that we'd been with at the Officer's Club, or they were our friends. It was a tremendously emotional experience. We just never knew who they were going to bring in next."[4]

Surgery personnel were divided into teams, each consisting of a lead surgeon, one other physician, one nurse, and one medic. All eight operating tables were filled within seconds of being emptied. Wooden sawhorses of uneven height were placed between the eight operating tables and used for litters to hold patients suffering from shock. With their feet higher than their heads, the patients' blood would drain quickly from the legs to the heart, which pumped it to their blood-deprived brains. Stacks of hot water bottles and blankets were kept near the sawhorses so that those suffering from shock could be made warm as rapidly as possible.

Because there was no electric sterilizer, steel-jacketed pressure cookers were placed over Bunsen burners to sterilize hundreds of pounds of surgical instruments, operating room gowns, gauze, towels, and swabs. These items were also sterilized in the utility room of the operating room. Circulating nurses sorted the newly sterilized items, stacking gowns, gauze, and linen into neat piles and placing surgical instruments on a large table covered by a sterile sheet. The instruments were then placed on smaller stands by each operating table as they were needed. In one thirty-six-hour period in January the surgical teams performed 425 major operations.

The American and Filipino forces were fighting against insurmountable odds. The lack of ammunition, equipment, and food created a horrendous potential for mounting numbers of dead and wounded. Gen. Jonathan Wainwright observed that in the long days and nights of the withdrawal from the north his original force of twenty-eight thousand men had been cut to about sixteen thousand, and they were in pitiable condition to start the ultimate defense of the Philippines.[5]

All the nurses on Bataan worked feverishly and without complaining, but Lieutenant Nash went beyond even this total dedication to duty. She had the respect and awe of all operating room personnel, because she seemed to be everywhere at once, making sure all surgical teams had the equipment they needed to give every wounded soldier the best chance for survival.

Capt. Alfred A. Weinstein, who practiced medicine in Atlanta before he joined the Army Medical Corps, recalled two of the nurses in the operating room of Hospital No.1. "Miss Frances Nash and Miss Easterling, two of our nurses, drove themselves as if beset by devils until their neatly starched uniforms were crumpled, sweat-soaked rags. Frances especially was a dynamo, driving the medics with her lashing tongue until they cussed her sullenly under their breath—not openly, because they were sure they'd get the back of her hand. A strapping, brown-haired, comely girl, raised on Georgia-grown pork, black eyed peas, hominy and grits, she packed a mean wallop."[6]

In addition to battle casualties, hundreds, then thousands of American and Filipino troops suffered from malaria, dengue or "break bone" fever, lack of food, and dysentery brought on by the absence of an uncontaminated water supply for front-line troops. Allied soldiers already acclimated to the tropical heat of Manila found they had never experienced anything like the heat and humidity of Bataan. Perspiration soaked through clothes in minutes and sweat ran constantly into one's eyes, blurring vision and necessitating almost continuous wiping and blotting to see clearly. Troops, nurses, and medical personnel fought and worked in unending clouds of dust that stuck to their sweat-soaked skin and made breathing in the hellish heat even more difficult. Despite the heat, soldiers frequently wore gas masks as protection against the dust that coated their bodies and left them looking like grayish-white creatures who had stumbled from the ocean's depths and lost their way.

Troops on the line suffered so drastically from thirst that they would drink from muddy and contaminated buffalo wallows or anywhere else they could find water. Individuals might last weeks without food, but Bataan's sizzling temperatures and lack of water would drive a person insane in thirty-six to forty-eight hours. The price of sanity in many jungle foxholes was amebic and bacillary dysentery. Troops too ill to be effective in fighting the Japanese were brought by the truckloads to Limay.

Nurses and medics who cared for these patients contracted dysentery in addition to the mosquito-borne malaria and dengue fever that already ravaged their weary bodies with headaches, rashes, nausea, vomiting, and temperatures of 104 or 105 degrees. Even though they fell prey to the same illnesses that had hospitalized their patients, nurses and doctors were on duty unless absolutely unable to perform their assignments.

Outside of surgery, the normal nursing routine consisted of a twelve- to twenty-hour day in which nurses reported to the wards at sunup. After an hour or so they were given a short break for a breakfast of tea and rice, then returned to their patients. The second and final meal for the day was served at 1600, and again nurses returned to their duties on the wards.

The job of ward nurse was literally backbreaking work. Patients' cots were approximately twelve inches off the floor, and the nurses had to bend over the patients to administer medical and postoperative treatments. Hour after hour of such work left nurses unable to straighten up without severe back and neck pain. No sooner would a nurse finish changing dressings on a ward than it was time to begin giving medications. After dark the nurses frequently carried flashlights in their mouths to leave their hands free for work. Hattie Brantley recalled those times: "I can remember doing dressings starting at breakfast and continuing through the day. I'd not go far along that line of cots before my back would not straighten up, and I'd get down on my knees, finally not even bothering to arise, but crawling to the next cot. My experience in a cotton patch back in East Texas stood me in good stead for this operation."[7]

Dressings were growing scarce as casualties increased and almost no new supplies arrived. To get as much use out of a dressing as possible, nurses would wash them out, dry them, and use them again for the next patient. The process was a never-ending circle.

During the second week in January 1942, rations were cut in half for the medical personnel as well as the troops on the battlefield. The number of casualties arriving at Hospital No.1 doubled. Morphine was one of the chief means of alleviating pain until the wounded could be treated. Nurses would fill a glass syringe with twenty doses of morphine and move from patient to patient, injecting them with the same needle, wiping the needle with alcohol after each use. The less than desirable conditions on Bataan made preparing to administer morphine no quick and easy task. Nurses had to sharpen needles on a rock or piece of stone, then boil the glass syringe and needle in water. When the glass syringe was considered sterile, morphine tablets were placed inside it, the needle connected, and the boiled water poured into the syringe to dissolve the morphine. This time-consuming procedure had to be followed for every twenty injections given to patients.

As January wore on, medications and dressings were becoming depleted. Quinine tablets were almost gone, and it was necessary to battle malaria with liquid quinine. The liquid had a bitter, astringent taste that added to the general suffering of troops and medical personnel. The morphine that had to be administered liberally to battle casualties was dwindling at an alarming rate, and ether, vitally needed for surgical procedures, was growing more scarce every day.

In late January 1942, the Japanese had progressed to the Moron-Bagac road and a battle ensued. When General Wainwright was ordered by General MacArthur to withdraw his forces to a reserve battle position, a midpoint of the Bataan peninsula that paralleled the Pilar-Bagac road, the fighting came within fifteen miles of Hospital No.1. More and more shells were flying overhead, and the Japanese had begun strafing the hospital. A decision was made to move the hospital compound from Limay to Little Baguio, a spot in the Bataan jungle approximately five miles south of Hospital No.2. Doctors and nurses spent two days placing plaster casts on fractured bones of the orthopedic patients so they could be transported. The day after Hospital No.1 was evacuated from Limay, Japanese bombers and artillery leveled the compound to the ground.

On Christmas Day 1941, twenty nurses left Manila on the SS *Hyde* to establish Hospital No.2 at Cabcaben, Bataan, under the command of Colonel Vanderboget. When 2d. Lt. Frances Nash was transferred on 26 December to Hospital No.1, the nurses who started Hospital No.2 were known as the "Original Nineteen." 2d. Lt. Josephine Nesbit, who was stationed on Corregidor, had one objection to her new assignment. "I was notified to be ready to take over as Chief Nurse of Bataan General Hospital No.2," Nesbit said. "I immediately complained that, if they wanted me to assume all that responsibility, they must promote me to 1st Lt. . . . Orders were cut at once for my assignment . . . as a 1st Lt . . . and I left the same day for the front lines of Bataan."[8]

The conditions there were primitive, and the nurses of Hospital No.2 were forced to bathe and wash their laundry in a nearby stream. For approximately ten days, some of the nurses slept on Pambusco buses, then it was decided that these buses, gathered in one area, presented a likely target for Japanese planes flying overhead. The buses were returned to the motor pool, and the nurses slept on cots under the trees.

The site selected for the hospital was approximately ten miles from the coastal village of Mariveles and the previously active Mariveles Naval Base on the southeast shore of Bataan. Since the only way into the site was by a narrow trail, army engineers used a bulldozer to cut a road and clear the site so that casualties could be delivered to and treated at the new field hospital. Medical supplies had been stored near the site before the war, and before the road was completed, equipment and supplies had to be carried by enlisted men from the storage dump to the hospital.

The mission of Hospital No.2 was to treat medical cases and the overflow of surgical patients from Hospital No.1. Since the hospital contained no buildings, several small tents, each holding six patients, were used for the most critically ill. By 9 January 1942, the number of casualties being cared for at Hospital No.2 had mushroomed. A decision was made to expand the hospital and a bulldozer was used to clear a large patch of jungle. Pieces of canvas and thatched mats were placed on the ground to serve as cots for the growing number of wounded.

1st Lt. Josie Nesbit remembered those days and one nurse in particular. "There was a sweet little nurse with me named Sally Blaine. I'd have to open a new ward just about every two days, and I'd say, 'Sally, I want you to go and open up that ward. Get it ready for another set of patients that are coming in.' I think she must have opened about ten wards for me. She said, 'What's the matter that you're making me do it?' I said, 'Sally, I can depend on you to do it right.' And she always did."[9]

Except for the operating room tent, the only overhead protection for the patients was the lush tropical foliage of jungle trees. Nurses and medical personnel worried about what would happen to their patients when the monsoon season started in May. The lack of protection created some unsettling experiences for the nurses, particularly those on night duty. Lt. Rita G. Palmer, a twenty-three-year-old native of Hampton, New Hampshire, recalled one of the hazards of night duty: "One of the nurses, I think it was Blanch Kimble, while making her rounds with a flashlight [got] hit solidly in the forehead. Putting her light up, she discovered that it was a snake swinging on a branch above. It had just hit her hard, which did not add to her peace of mind for the rest of that night."[10]

By 23 January thirty-four Filipina and thirteen army nurses had been transferred from Hospital No.1 to Hospital No.2 to help care for the wounded troops. As in Hospital No.1, nurses in Hospital No.2 suffered from malaria, dengue fever, dysentery, and inadequate food. Spurred by a clear purpose and determination to care for sick and wounded troops, nurses did what they could to keep themselves going and continued to care for their patients.

After weeks without any protection from mosquitoes, Hospital No.2 received mosquito nets for individual cots. They were welcomed by the nurses, who quickly had them set up for patients and medical personnel. Nurses soon learned, however, that the nets were a mixed blessing. Lieutenant Nesbit reported: "One night in the dark, someone was yelling at the top of her lungs. I stumbled through the dark toward the screams. I thought maybe a Jap had gotten through. I was relieved to discover that a big rat had gotten in bed with one of the nurses and was trapped by the mosquito netting until she could pull it free, and the rat could run back into the underbrush of our jungle home."[11]

As the Battle of Bataan wore on, more and more cases of gas gangrene were admitted to Hospital No.2. The spores that caused this life-threatening condition lived in Bataan's tropical soil, which was rich with anaerobic bacteria such as Bacillus Welshii (now known as *Clostridium perfringens*). In the absence of oxygen, this bacteria proliferated rapidly in muscles damaged by deep, perforating wounds. The bacillus formed tiny bubbles in and around the injured tissue and exerted pressure on blood vessels, cutting off the flow of oxygen to the wound and resulting in the death of tissue and muscle. The bacteria also formed a toxin that traveled along nerve trunks to the brain, causing death in as few as three days. Amputations of infected arms and legs were performed routinely in hopes of stopping the bacteria before its toxin could travel its lethal journey through the nervous system. Many who escaped this horrible death faced the rest of their lives with one leg or one arm.

Since casualties could be transported only at night, wounded troops frequently had to wait eighteen to twenty-four hours for anything more than rudimentary first aid. This delay was responsible for a sharp increase in the number of gas gangrene cases transferred from Hospital No.1. Before these patients were transferred, Hospital No.2 had had no gas gangrene infections, and to help stem the rise in these cases, patients were treated in a ward set apart from the rest of the hospital. Because sulfathiazide powder was all but depleted and the supply of antitoxin developed during World War I had long been exhausted, another method had to be found to treat this contagious and frequently fatal infection.

A method of treatment barely explored with gas gangrene patients in World War I was enlarged upon by Colonel Adamo, a Filipino army physician, who was assigned to Hospital No.2. He put this treatment into practice in the army hospitals on Bataan. The process involved opening and enlarging the wound and exposing the infection to the oxygen and sunlight that were the deadly enemies of Bacillus Welchii. The effect of this treatment was dramatic. As Dr. Alfred Weinstein said: "In many instances the soldiers lost their toxicity in twelve to twenty-four hours. Their pulses slowed, their blood pressure rose, they lost their mental confusion, and they took nourishment.... If they were worse in twenty-four hours, it became necessary, in an attempt to save life, to consider amputating a leg, leaving the cut exposed to the air." [12]

As illness and battle wounds increased, the food supply for all American and Filipino troops on Bataan dwindled. The military retreated farther and farther into the Bataan peninsula, driving carabao ahead of it. Carabao meat augmented the food supply while the beasts lasted. The meat was tough and had a strong taste. Different recipes were tried to make the meat more palatable, but no matter how long the meat was cooked, it never lost the tough, enduring quality of a well-made shoe. One recipe for cooking carabao was well known to marines and soldiers alike. Lt. Col. William E. Dyess remembered it well: "Place the carabao meat in a pot of boiling water with a large rock. When the rock melts, the carabao is done." [13]

Canned fruit, vegetables, milk, rice, beans, flour, coffee, and cocoa were supplemented by whatever food could be bought or hunted. In December and partway through January medical personnel were able to buy some poultry and eggs from nearby village farmers.

Dr. Weinstein depicted one of these food hunts in his book *Barbed-Wire Surgeon*:

> I went foraging, buying as much food as I could in the provincial capital of Balanea, north of us, and stored as much as I could in my car.... The day before Christmas, Gus and I drove along a narrow dusty road looking for food. Thoughts of my last Christmas in Atlanta, spiced with the taste of Southern-fried chicken, candied yams

and marshmallows and Brunswick stew, flitted through
my mind when we saw a sign, "Chickens for Sale. . . ." On
the outskirts of the jungle we were shown a model
chicken farm. Hundreds of plump Plymouth Rocks and
Rhode Island Reds in wire coops elevated from the
ground, lined the yard that was immaculately clean.

"I am Jose Guenena. I am a graduate of an agricultural
school, Sir," the Filipino said proudly. "And now my fat
birds will be killed by bombs or eaten by the Japs."

The price was right—a dollar a bird, a half buck for a
fryer.[14]

The chicken was a welcomed recognizable meat. Not all meat
was so clearly defined by the palate. Dr. Weinstein remembered
one instance with his characteristic vividness: "One day we were
served a meat stew which had an especially strong flavor and
unchewable quality. 'Is this beef, Sergeant Moreno?' I asked.

'No, Sir.'

'It doesn't taste like carabao. Is it?'

'No, Sir.'

'What the hell is it?'

'Twenty-seventh cavalry, Sir,' he said sadly."[15]

Meat from mules, donkeys, and horses was served to supplement the diet as food supplies began to disappear. Many thorough-
bred horses, including a favorite mount of General Wainwright's,
were eventually served as food to the troops that had ridden and
cared for them.

As conditions became more desperate on Bataan, monkeys,
previously treated as pets in the camps, began to disappear from
their accustomed places. Snakes and lizards were no longer seen as
pests or possible enemies but as sources of protein. They were served
up at mess and in foxholes as other foodstuffs became scarce. In
March the food ration, cut in half in January, was cut in half again
for all American and Filipino troops on Bataan.

In early March, when Japanese general Masaharu Homma
landed more troops in the Lingayen Gulf area, he increased the

Japanese force on Bataan to 250,000. Along with the infusion of Japanese troops came a written demand for the surrender of Bataan. General Wainwright reported: "The demand was dropped from planes over Bataan. It was dropped in thousands of empty beer cans, to each of which was attached red and white ribbons to make spotting easier." [16]

The Allied forces numbered about seventy thousand men; many were not combat troops, and they were in poor condition. Supplies of every kind were disappearing as the Japanese fought their way down the peninsula. Nurses and medical personnel now ate one meal a day and were determined to care for their patients even if the food ration was cut again. As March drew to a close, the chief nurse, Josie Nesbit, called the nurses together to tell them that the food supply was almost gone. "We've got to make what we have, last. If necessary we'll have one meal every two days. I know you won't complain." [17]

The nurses found it easier to do without food than to respond to some of the questions of wounded soldiers, some barely out of their teens. Questions ranged from "Am I going to make it?" to "What will happen to us if help doesn't come?" Nurses and doctors debated among and with themselves the morality of telling a dying patient that he was going to live. Was it better for the soldier to know he was dying so he could prepare his soul for death, or was it better for him not to know, even be reassured that he was going to recover?

Dr. Weinstein spoke for most medical personnel when he said: "The argument raged back and forth with nobody knowing the correct answer. Most of us followed a middle course, ducking the question or avoiding a direct answer. If a patient looked as if he might kick the bucket, we called in the chaplain to give him last rites, collect personal mementos, and write last messages. Their appearance meant to the wounded that they were seriously ill, yet did not have the same disastrous mental effect of a fiat. . . . More often than not, they didn't have to be told. As days wore on and they steadily became weaker, they adjusted themselves to the fact that they were not going to live." [18]

The indomitable human spirit was always evident among the nurses, doctors, medical personnel, and troops. A large part of that unconquerable spirit was the ability to laugh in the face of fear and the horrors of war. The nurses who served on Bataan and Corregidor and were prisoners of war in the Philippines were quick to point out that "without a sense of humor, people just shriveled up and died." A sense of humor went far in getting nurses through the countless numbers of casualties who needed their help and the wounded who were beyond their help. As 2d Lt. Juanita Redmond noted regarding the tragedy and the humor experienced in war, "The things you want to forget and the things you hope you'll remember are all inextricably mixed up together."[19] Humor was a vital part of the human spirit that created and affirmed camaraderie among the defenders of the Philippines and those who survived more than three years of Japanese internment. Events like those described below helped break the indescribable tension that filled every day in the hospitals on Bataan and later on Corregidor.

Lt. Frances Nash related an incident that occurred during the long hours of continuous surgery. While they were in the operating room, a gas attack warning broke the silence of eight operating teams intent on their lifesaving work. "Everyone pulled his mask up and over his face. Helmets and gas masks were a must at all times in surgery. All of a sudden a fine surgeon from Atlanta put his hands up, cursing in Yiddish. I closed in at his back and whispered. 'What's wrong?' He said, 'I'm a blind surgeon!!' I said, 'Did you check your mask, tell me the truth.' He replied, 'No.' He took it off and I pulled out the original cardboard and packing so he could see. Dead silence in [the] pavilion—but I heard a lot of ribbing from the doctors went on later."[20]

On the first night Nash arrived on Bataan, casualties streamed into the operating room. Surgeons, physicians, and corpsmen were brought in to render assistance to the wounded. At this point new faces were not unusual as medical personnel were brought in under War Plan Orange 3 from all posts in the Philippines to work on the newest lines of defense. Nor was it unusual in time of war to remove the insignia of rank from all uniforms so as not to provide a tempting target for enemy snipers, who might find the target of a lieutenant, captain, or major irresistible.

Despite the confusion of the overflowing surgical unit, where two hundred casualties were lined up and waiting, Lieutenant Nash was supervising with an eagle eye. She related the following incident:

> A Navy man was doing an excellent job supplying the tables with sterile instruments and we were doing fine. All of a sudden he said, "Get me a sterile saw, clamps and sutures on a tray, quick! I'll get ready to take this leg off."
>
> I said, "Oh, no you will not, get back to doing your job. In the Army we don't practice on the wounded."
>
> He rushed out back to the C.O. who returned and introduced the Commander as a surgeon. I didn't know he was a surgeon. He had no uniform insignia.
>
> The Commander later used to look back at me. I would walk up behind the surgeons and they could tell me if they were in trouble and see if I could get what they needed. He would smile, whisper, "Boss, just wanted to know if I could operate."[21]

One night at Hospital No.2, a storm was approaching, and strong winds were blowing dust and whipping through the trees when Lieutenant Redmond decided to move several gas gangrene patients into the cover of a small shed she had had cleaned to give them shelter. She directed all the corpsmen who could be spared to carry those patients, in their beds, from the open ward to the shed. Since they were working in total darkness, Redmond directed her flashlight beam toward the ground to prevent the corpsmen from falling over rocks and tree roots. Suddenly the occupant of one of the beds in transit sat upright.

> "What the hell's going on here?" he shouted. The next instant he jumped out and started to run.
>
> "Don't run, don't run," I called in an agony of anxiety. "Wait, we'll take you in."

I turned my flashlight on him, and recognized one of the corpsmen. "Well," I said furiously, "what in the name of Pete were you doing in that bed, Caston?"

The corpsman explained, while trying to cover his bare legs with his too short shirttails, that he had been so tired when he got off duty, he simply sank into an empty bed and fell asleep. "You get your trousers and help us move the other patients," Redmond ordered. Caston followed her orders without a complaint despite the fact that he was officially off duty.[22]

As April began, Hospital No.2 stretched for more than two and a half miles and had more than seven thousand sick and wounded soldiers in the care of seventy-eight military and Filipina nurses, with new casualties arriving by the hundreds every day. In some wards, foxholes had been dug directly under patients' cots so the wounded could be afforded as much protection as possible should the hospital be shelled or bombed. It was now patently clear to all but the delusional that help was not going to arrive in time to prevent their deaths or eventual capture by the enemy.

On 8 April 1942 General Wainwright's troops were attacked by heavy Japanese bombers. He made arrangements to move battalions from Bataan to Corregidor and to move the nurses to Mariveles for evacuation. These personnel would be crucial for the defense of the Rock. At 2200 on the night of 8 April, the nurses were told that they were being evacuated to Corregidor immediately and that General Edward P. King Jr. would surrender Bataan at 0600 the following day. All nurses were to report to trucks and buses waiting to transport them to Mariveles with only what they could carry in their two hands.

The hospital at Little Baguio became the new site of Hospital No.1. Before war broke out in the Philippines, this area was used as a motor pool by troops on maneuvers. Now it would house nurses, doctors, medical personnel, and patients. A deep artesian well was located on a hill overlooking the hospital half a mile away. In addition, there was a large concrete pool that could be used to chlorinate the hospital's water supply. Water was run by gravity to the hospital site. The hospital compound was about two acres in size, fringed by hardwood trees and swept by cool breezes. The site was surrounded on three sides by potential enemy targets: to the north, ammunition dumps; to the south, the quartermaster food dump; and to the east, the engineer's supply dump. There were six concrete-floored, tin-roofed sheds that had been used as garages before the Battle of Bataan began. Additional sheds of similar construction were built around the compound, increasing the bed capacity to a thousand.

A wooden frame building stood in the center of the compound. It was similar in size to the surgical area at Hospital No.1, and in a day, Frances Nash and her crew had it cleaned and organized as Little Baguio's surgical pavilion. In the rear of the compound were two large wooden structures that were used for an officers' quarters and a nurses' quarters with a combined officers' mess. Engineers installed electrical wiring, lights, and indoor plumbing.

When Hospital No.1 and the combat troops moved toward the southern tip of Bataan, the Japanese apparently decided to give their army a rest. For about ten days, there was a welcomed lull in the fighting, which resulted in a drastic reduction of casualties. Nurses, doctors, and medical personnel had a chance to relax and think of something other than war and its carnage. A swimming party was arranged at Siseman Cove on the coast, facing Corregidor. Four Allied PT boats floated several hundred yards off shore. Nurses, doctors, and medical personnel changed their clothes, ran happily down the sloping beach, and splashed into the warm tropical water of Manila Bay. They swam and played in the water, then returned to shore to eat carabao sandwiches and to share a fruit drink made of native limes which grew liberally in the area. Toward the end of the day, they drove back to Little Baguio feeling rested and refreshed.

During this lull in the battle, romances begun in Manila blossomed again along with some social activities. The commanding officer gave his permission for a dance to be held in the officers' mess. An old hand-cranked portable phonograph and fifteen or twenty records, all from the 1920s, provided the music. This opportunity afforded overworked personnel with much needed relaxation and diversion from their daily labors.

The next day an army truck driver brought the news that the Japanese were on the move again. Hand-to-hand combat was now taking place between Allied frontline troops and the Japanese. Ammunition was gone. Soldiers brought to the hospital were hungry, dehydrated, and suffering from exhaustion and the loss of blood. They had lain in their foxholes for days before being transported to the hospital at Little Baguio.

The horrors of battle and lack of basic supplies were intensified by the fanaticism with which the enemy on Bataan fought. The Japanese soldier stood in stark contrast to American and Filipino troops. The militaristic history and philosophy of Bushido turned every soldier into a killer determined to win for the emperor at all costs. The lives of Japanese soldiers were valued cheaply by their officers and emperor alike. According to Bushido, a Japanese soldier who was captured or surrendered had disgraced himself and his entire family. Ritualistic suicide, hari kari, was ingrained into the ranks and command of the empire of Japan. Soldiers, taught that they would be tortured and enslaved if taken prisoners, fought with little or no thought of their own survival. This philosophy caused the Japanese soldiers to hold in contempt any captured enemy or prisoner of war and led them to inflict the most brutal atrocities on enemy troops. It was not uncommon for overrun or captured Allied troops to be found with their hands tied behind their backs, their bodies riddled with scores of bayonet wounds.

Americans and Filipinos learned quickly to recognize the beginning of a major Japanese offensive. Driven by the code of Bushido, the attack would begin with the sounds of machine-gun fire, followed in rapid succession by waves of screaming Japanese shock troops who threw themselves willingly upon land mines that exploded beneath them and scattered their bodies along the front of the charge. Hundreds of their comrades then ran across their torn bodies toward Filipino and American troops. The Bushido-driven sacrifice would continue as Japanese soldiers hurled themselves into electrified barbed-wire, pulling it to the ground. Their comrades used their bodies as bridges to close with Allied troops and engage in hand-to-hand combat. The smell of death and decaying bodies permeated the hot, dust-filled air of the peninsula.

Adding to this horror were hundreds of Japanese snipers who made their way behind enemy lines, climbed into trees, tied themselves to the branches, and shot at combat troops, wounded soldiers, nurses, and medical personnel. They brought death in unexpected places, magnifying the horror of war by nullifying any and all "safety zones." Allied troops were forced to fire into treetops, hoping to hit an enemy who used smokeless powder to conceal his position.

When night fell, the snipers who were still alive would untie themselves, climb down from their perches of death, and sneak back into their own lines. Hundreds of dead snipers were left behind, their bodies suspended in treetops to swell and rot in the insufferable heat. For every Japanese soldier the Allies killed, there were hundreds more to replace them.

A separate ward was constructed for Japanese wounded and surrounded by barbed-wire, more to keep vengeful Filipinos out than to keep the Japanese in. The Japanese patients received the same linen, food, and cigarette issue as American wounded. Dr. Weinstein described those Japanese patients: "Exsanguinated, begrimed, with massive wounds covered with dirt and maggots, most of them were too weak to resist our attempts to clean, feed and operate on them. After the first few days of sullen terror, the Japanese patients finally got it through their thick skulls that we were trying to heal them."[23]

It was not easy for American and Filipina nurses and doctors to treat Japanese casualties in the same manner as they treated their own sick and wounded. None had ever heard of an American or Filipino soldier being given aid by the Japanese. Frances Nash spoke of these facts with a mixture of sadness and anger: "American medics brought Jap wounded to us. We let them keep all the American socks, underwear and watches they had lined up on their wrists. Made you want to say something bad when you saw the laundry mark on a garment of someone's name you knew. It meant the person was dead."[24]

One of the first things nurses and medical personnel did when they reached the compound at Little Baguio and established the hospital was to spread white sheets in the form of a cross along the side of the hill near the hospital wards. They hoped the Japanese would respect the noncombatant hospital site and not shell or bomb it. Those hopes were dashed when at 1000 on 30 March 1942, Japanese planes bombed the hospital and scored a direct hit in the compound. Fourteen native bed makers were killed and a truck loaded with dead, charred bodies lay on its side in the road. Hospital corpsman Pfc. Fred Lang was brought in dead with a hole through his heart. Another medic, M.Sgt. Spielhoffer, was carried in with one of his feet torn off. He would die later of an uncontrolled infection.

Dr. Weinstein remembered a Japanese broadcast after the bombing. "'We regret the unfortunate bombing of hospital. It was a mistake.' We knew it was deliberate. We knew we were living on borrowed time."[25]

On 6 April 1942, the day after Easter, Japanese bombers returned to Little Baguio to bomb the hospital again. This time a foxhole filled with Filipino mess attendants was hit and the Filipinos were crushed to death by falling debris. Less than an hour later, Japanese planes returned to bomb the hospital again. The pilot scored a direct hit, and a half-ton bomb landed in the center of a ward. The bomb killed 100 patients and medical personnel and injured another 150. Bodies were blown into the branches of trees, and pieces of bodies were everywhere. The sound of the plane's engines was replaced by the screams, moans, and weeping of the newly wounded.

Frances Nash remembered the carnage and her anger at the Japanese: "In that raid several wards were wiped out completely. One of them contained thirty or more head cases, boys without eyes, ears or noses. I had never before been so mad at any individual that I wanted to kill him, as I did the Japs. I was so mad that I wasn't frightened."[26]

Surviving the raid was only half the battle. Surviving the bomb's aftermath was more difficult in many ways. Images of dismembered bodies and the sounds of fear, horror, and pain were burned into the memories of those who witnessed the ravages of war, a glimpse into hell.

In her book *I Served on Bataan*, Lt. Juanita Redmond described the scene in unforgettable words: "There were mangled bodies under the ruins; a bloodstained hand stuck up through a pile of scrap; arms and legs had been ripped off and flung among the rubbish. Some of the mangled torsos were almost impossible to identify. One of the few medics who had survived unhurt climbed a tree to bring down a body blown into the top branches. We were shaking and sick to our stomachs, but none of us who was able to go on dared to stop even for a moment."[27]

During this raid two nurses, 2d Lts. Rosemary Hogan and Rita Palmer, were wounded and required surgical attention. Hogan was wounded in the face and shoulder, Palmer in the chest and leg. The latter said: "I remember coming to and having, you know, long beams of the roof over me and struggling out from under those . . . somebody helped. I don't know who. . . . And I didn't know about the place on [in] my chest for several hours. . . . It's [shrapnel] in my chest cavity and every time I have an x-ray, it's in a different place. . . . In my leg, I have little pieces of shrapnel . . . nothing that's really debilitating."[28]

Only sixty-five beds of the original sixteen hundred in the field hospital at Little Baguio were still standing. All patients except those too ill to be moved were transferred to Hospital No.2. Rosemary Hogan and Rita Palmer were transferred to Corregidor for further medical treatment of their wounds.[29]

One of the many items in short supply on Bataan was clothing. Large numbers of American and Filipino soldiers were fighting in shreds and swatches of their original uniforms. To provide the living with better clothes, uniforms in relatively good condition were stripped from the dead and distributed among frontline troops.

At Little Baguio the burial of the dead was supervised by the chaplains. Bodies were stored until night, when enlisted men accompanied the chaplains to a place in the jungle, away from the hospital wards. A bulldozer was used to dig a common grave because the numbers of dead grew every day. One of the dead soldier's identification tags was left on the body, the other brought back to the hospital to be kept and used to establish accurate records.

One evening, Lt. Frances Nash walked out to the new burial site to collect the identification tags and any clothes that might have been overlooked. Although she had seen thousands of wounded and dying soldiers, the common grave site had a strong and lasting effect on her: "I never went back again. Too much for me, got to thinking I may be next."[30]

On 8 April 1942 the Allies' line north of the hospitals broke, and the Japanese pushed within three miles of the medical facilities. The patients and staff were in grave danger; some American and Filipino soldiers were seen retreating on foot toward the southern tip of Bataan. That night, orders to evacuate to Corregidor were delivered to Colonel Duckworth from General Wainwright's headquarters on Corregidor.

When Chief Nurse Nesbit learned the Filipina nurses were not included in the evacuation, she protested and told her superior, Colonel J.D. Gillespie, M.D., that she would stay on Bataan with them. "I was adamant about this matter because some of these same Japanese troops were also the perpetrators and were responsible for the 'Rape of Nanking,' China . . . in 1937. I did not want this fate to befall our own women, whether Americans or Filipinas."[31]

As a result of Lieutenant Nesbit's insistence, General Wainwright hurriedly amended his orders to include the hospitals' Filipina nurses. Colonel Duckworth ordered that all of the nurses were to be evacuated to Corregidor. They were given five minutes to report to the buses that would carry them to the docks at Mariveles and told to bring only what they could carry in their hands. Bataan would be surrendered at 0600 the following day. The nurses refused to leave their patients and had to be given a direct order to evacuate to Corregidor to care for the sick and wounded on the Rock.

Navy nurses who were already prisoners of war were caring for wounded and sick patients. On 10 January 1942 the five navy nurses captured on Guam in December were placed aboard the Japanese ship *Argentina Maru* and, along with captured marines and sailors, were taken to the island of Shikoku in southern Japan and placed in Zentsuji prison camp.

On 8 March 1942, the eleven navy nurses held in Santa Scholastica were placed in cars and driven the approximately two miles to the civilian internment camp at Santo Tomas.

5

From the Frying Pan into the Fire

*Never forget the American girls who fought on Bataan and
later on Corregidor. . . . The memory of their coming ashore
on Corregidor that early morning of April 9, dirty, dishev-
eled, some of them wounded from the hospital bombings—
and every last one of them with her chin up in the air—is a
memory that can never be erased.*

Gen. Jonathan M. Wainwright

Hunger, disease, and combat had been taking their toll on American and Filipino troops for months. More than eight thousand sick
and wounded patients covered the ground under jungle trees at
Hospital No. 2 and Little Baguio. Medical personnel and troops
were just about out of medicines, bandages, food, ammunition,
and able-bodied men—in fact they were just about out of everything except wounded and sick soldiers. When General King decided to surrender Bataan as of 9 April, he ordered the evacuation
of nurses and many troops to Corregidor, where they would make
their last stand.

The two field hospitals on Bataan were approximately five miles
apart, and they received word of the surrender only hours ahead of
the advancing Japanese who were fighting their way down the peninsula. The nurses left for Mariveles in different groups and by alter-
nate routes. Those at Hospital No. 2 had a longer distance to travel,
and the way was clogged with vehicles, soldiers, and civilians.

The nurses were filled with a myriad of emotions, including feelings of guilt and sorrow at leaving their patients and the doctors and corpsmen with whom they had worked so closely since 8 December, when the Japanese attacked the Philippines. It had been difficult enough to see men who had been their friends, their military families, torn apart by strafing, bombing, bullets, and shells. It was almost unbearable now to leave these men vulnerable and defenseless, their patients, their friends and co-workers, and to move to the relative, temporary safety of Corregidor. A few of the nurses, like Denny Williams, were leaving their sick, hospitalized soldier-husbands.

Lt. Maude "Denny" Williams received the order that the nurses must leave in thirty minutes. She had already been told that the Japanese were within three miles of Hospital No.2 and pushing steadily forward. She grabbed her musette bag, placed all the quinine she had left inside it, picked up a canteen of water, and headed for the officers' ward. Although they had been ordered not to tell the patients that they were leaving, Denny could not keep the truth from her husband. "We're leaving," she said. "Bill, I don't want to go." Her husband was quick to point out that ordering the nurses to leave meant Bataan was going to be surrendered, and Denny surely had to get out. She gave him the quinine and canteen. "Take care of yourself for my sake," she said. They kissed good-bye and Denny left.[1]

They went reluctantly, under a direct order that had to be repeated to army nurses who had been taught, and believed to their core, that nurses did not leave their patients and that military nurses did not leave wounded soldiers, sailors, and marines for the sake of their own safety. The direct order was repeated again, not for reasons of the nurses' safety but based on the cold, hard fact that the wounded and sick on Corregidor, where the military's last stand would·be made, would need the specialized care that these nurses could provide.

Lt. Hattie Brantley was among the nurses at Little Baguio who received orders at sundown on 8 April to pack a musette bag and board an old army bus to begin their evacuation to Corregidor. The doctors and other medical personnel stood around and joked with the nurses as they reluctantly climbed onto the bus that was to carry them to Mariveles, a small town on the southern tip of Bataan. "They said things like 'The Golden Gate in '48!' and 'Help is on the way!'" Brantley said.[2]

The bus moved out at a snail's pace, carrying the nurses through a scene of chaotic activity. The army was blowing up ammunition dumps on all sides, and fires from the explosions bathed the night sky with an eerie light. Shells from Corregidor's guns were roaring overhead as vehicles jammed the roads and soldiers slogged along in thick clouds of dust. Civilians pounded on both sides of the bus and begged to be taken on board. Nurses were forced to close their eyes and ears to these pleas to be taken along with the evacuating military. "If we had taken one and not another," Brantley said, "there would have been a riot and none of us would have gotten through. But God, it was hard!"[3]

Nurses who had gotten off duty and gone to bed were awakened and hurried into vehicles for the evacuation to Mariveles and Corregidor. Lt. Geneva Jenkins, a thirty-one-year-old Tennessean, was sound asleep when she received word of the evacuation. "I had gone to bed after laundering all my clothes and had them stretched up on the line," Jenkins said. "They said, 'You have to leave.' So, here I ran off with all my underwear on the line."[4]

The car that carried Jenkins and other nurses was hit by shrapnel and stopped in the middle of the road. They got out and started walking. A truck came along and the driver recognized Jenkins as the nurse who had taken care of him in the Little Baguio hospital. He stopped, loaded the nurses on board, and drove them to the wharf at Mariveles, where they got on a boat that took them to Corregidor.

How the nurses traveled across Manila Bay to Corregidor depended largely on what time they reached Mariveles and what type of boat was available. "We were put on open barges," Nash said. "Lying flat on some coiled rope, I heard shrapnel falling in the bay all around me, and I hugged the deck tighter and tighter. It took from 9:10 P.M. that night, until 3:00 A.M. the next morning to make what had been a 30 minute run in peacetime."[5]

At one point during the evacuation, a soldier used a rowboat to take several nurses across the bay. A few nurses were left behind because the boat could not carry all of them at once. Jerry McDuval, the young soldier in charge of the rowboat, promised to return promptly for the others. As the rowboat pulled away from the dock, an army nurse from his hometown, Lockhart, Texas, called after him, "Jerome! If you don't come back and get me, I'm gonna tell your mama when I get home!"[6] As promised, the young man returned with a launch and evacuated the remaining nurses. Jerome's mother must have heard only good stories from Lt. Eunice Hatchitt.

The trip across Manila Bay was a nightmare. The bay was crowded with boats of all sizes, from rowboats to twenty-five-foot-long fishing boats. In between were homemade rafts and just about anything that would float. Some desperate soldiers and civilians were attempting to swim to Corregidor through the shark-infested water. As boats carrying the nurses made their way toward the Rock, they were engulfed in a cacophony of sounds. Japanese planes were bombing and strafing Manila Bay. The sound of the shrapnel made pitting noises as it struck the water and boats around them. Screams tore through the eerie darkness as people were hit or their boats were shot out from under them. Men and women in the water were crying for help, but it was impossible to stop. Each boat was already filled to capacity, and saving those in the water might well have meant the rescuing vessel and its passengers would also find themselves in the bay. Cries died out as people sank beneath the surface and drowned, and other desperate individuals took their places. For the nurses who had been ordered to leave their patients on Bataan, the scene was straight out of hell.

Not all the nurses arrived at Mariveles on the night of 8 April. One group from Hospital No. 2 did not reach the wharf until daylight the next morning. Officially Bataan surrendered at 0600, and no one, according to the rules of war, was supposed to leave the peninsula after the white flag went up. Lt. Minnie Breese related why the nurses were late arriving at Mariveles and some of the hazards they faced getting there:

> I was on night duty the night we were to be evacuated. They didn't say surrender the camp. They said we were all going to be taken to Corregidor.
>
> How can you leave a ward full of patients. . . . Those eyes just followed us. . . . I've always been a bedside nurse, and it's hard to leave your patients like that. So we hung on as long as we could, until they just forced us to go and get into the truck. Well, by that time, it was too late. Our troops were confused; they didn't know where to go. They were desperate. . . . Bataan is just a peninsula and you could hear the Japs up there hollering, "Bonzai!" and all that stuff that they chatter, and we could hear the firing of shells right over us. I was sick anyway that night. I had malaria and dysentery. Colonel North [doctor] told me to take . . . 30 grains of quinine. . . . We had a little bit left. Of course it made me deaf as a post and nauseated . . . I didn't care really if I lived or died. Well, I got on the truck, and Sally Durrett took care of me. . . . I remember vomiting and running behind the bush with dysentery.[7]

The truck they were traveling in had to stop because of exploding ammunition dumps. The nurses lay on the side of the road for about an hour watching shells and explosives brighten the night sky above Bataan's trees. When they finally reached the docks, the last boat had already left and daylight had come. Breese suggested that the group go to the navy tunnel where they might find food and water. When they reached the entrance, they discovered that the navy had blown up the tunnel rather than leave it for the Japanese.

The chief nurse, Lt. Josie Nesbit, finally got through to Corregidor by telephone and asked that a boat be sent to get her group off Bataan. "I remember when the boat arrived," Breese said. "I was so dizzy . . . I couldn't see straight. They said, 'Get on this plank.' I said, 'What plank?' I was so dizzy. That's when I lost all my clothes. I couldn't carry them in the suitcase. I was just so sick. Finally got in the boat . . . it was a little boat . . . and we finally got over to Corregidor."[8]

No one would forget the trip to reach the bay or the boat ride to the Rock. Along with the other horrors of war, the evacuation scene was indelibly burned into the nurses' memories.

6

![American flag]

The Tunnel and the Rock

I request that you convey the special commendation and gratitude of the War Department to the nurses of Corregidor whose service is a source of inspiration to all of us.

Gen. George C. Marshall, Army Chief of Staff,
in a message to General Wainwright, 18 April 1942

The second group of nurses arrived on Corregidor in daylight and in the midst of an air raid. The once beautiful green sloping lawns and trees of the tiny island had been transformed by Japanese bombs into charred stumps and denuded gray rock. In the coming weeks, enemy planes and artillery shells would pound away at the Rock, trying to dislodge its defenders and destroy the relative safety of the tunnel.

Malinta Tunnel was sunk deep into the rock that was Corregidor. Its main shaft ran east and west for 750 feet, and its center lay under more than 100 feet of concrete, rock, and vegetation, with an interior height of approximately 15 feet and a width of 25 feet. Branching from the main tunnel were twenty smaller tunnels, called laterals, which ran north to south. From one of these laterals, seven other branches ran parallel to the main tunnel, shallower than the Malinta and originally constructed for storage. These rooms became the hospital wards, nurses' quarters, doctors' quarters, and Gen. Jonathan Wainwright's headquarters and living area.

The north-south laterals housed various components of the fort such as quartermaster, machine shop, and refrigeration plant.

The hospital laterals were originally equipped to handle five hundred beds, but by the time of Corregidor's surrender on 6 May 1942, the hospital held fifteen hundred patients, housed in double- and triple-decked beds, built by the Rock's quartermaster and machine shop divisions.

After the horrors of Bataan, nurses welcomed the comparative safety of the tunnel. It would not be long, however, before Corregidor and Malinta Tunnel would become their own little corner of hell.

One main entrance to Malinta lay to the west and was wide enough to permit two ambulances, side by side, to enter the hospital lateral, where they were met by nurses and stretcher-bearers who would sort and carry the wounded to the appropriate wards and surgery. Nurses from Bataan were pleasantly surprised to find an enameled white table beside each of the five hundred beds and electric lights, bare bulbs, hanging from the ceiling of the Malinta and each of its laterals.

By 9 April 1942, when all nurses from Bataan had arrived in Malinta Tunnel, the forces defending Corregidor numbered 11,000. They were opposed by 250,000 Japanese.

In addition to military personnel, hundreds of civilians sought shelter in Malinta. The Japanese had allowed civilians through their lines knowing that these refugees would further deplete the military's food and water supplies and add to the crowded conditions in the tunnel. Nurses who had seen thousands of wounded, ill, and dying soldiers were now confronted with an increasing stream of hungry, exhausted, and sick refugees arriving every day. Many of them brought their children or children entrusted to them by relatives and friends. One orphaned six-year-old boy, suffering from malaria and wandering about Bataan, was found by soldiers and brought to Malinta Tunnel. The child was cared for by nurses who set up a bed for him in an old bathtub that was away from the wounded and dying in the regular hospital laterals. When the boy recovered from the attack of malaria, he continued to live in the tunnel and sleep in his bathtub bed, looked after by nurses, medical personnel, soldiers, and civilians. So that the child would not be left unattended while nurses were on almost twenty-four-hour duty, they arranged for the boy to spend much of his time with the Chinese tailor who worked in the tunnel, making uniforms to replace those that were quickly becoming rags.

In addition to the growing numbers of wounded soldiers and the decreasing supplies of medicines, bandages, anesthetics, water, and food, the tunnel presented its own unique set of problems. Malinta had been prepared in the 1920s as part of War Plan Orange 3 to serve as the final and impregnable fortress of Corregidor. Its planners believed that supplies could be brought in regularly by air and water and that Corregidor would never be conquered by an enemy. Therefore, the idea of having to surrender the Rock was never a question. None of the tunnel's organizers or the designers of War Plan Orange 3 had foreseen that control of the skies over the Philippines would be lost to the enemy in two to three days. Nor had they foreseen the fleet of Japanese warships that would cut off supplies by sea or the force of 250,000 Japanese troops, well fed, well supplied, and fresh with reinforcements, who would assail starving, exhausted, poorly equipped, wounded, and ill troops, who were eventually outnumbered approximately twenty-one to one. The tunnel had not been planned to hold the five thousand people who sought refuge inside its walls during air raids and artillery attacks that grew from frequent, to heavy, to constant as the Battle of Corregidor dragged on. As 2d Lt. Hattie R. Brantley put it: "The Japanese did not defeat us on Bataan and Corregidor. We were defeated by lack of food and medicines, and the abundance of sick and wounded patients."[1]

Nurses who had been ordered to leave their patients on Bataan and move to the Rock often wondered about the fate of those patients and American and Filipino troops left behind. The world would discover their fate when several soldiers who had survived the Bataan Death March escaped from prisoner of war camps and reached Allied lines. They brought news that shocked the military and the world, that wounded soldiers had been bayoneted in their cots or left to die of thirst. They also told of the atrocities visited on American and Filipino troops during the brutal march from Bataan to the Japanese POW camp at Camp O'Donnell. By July 1942, fourteen thousand Americans and Filipinos had died in Camp O'Donnell alone. One army air corps pilot, William Dyess, who escaped and related his story to General MacArthur, was told: "It is a story that should be told to the American people. But I am afraid, Captain, that the people back home will find it hard to believe you. I believe you. Make no mistake about that. I know the Japs."[2]

Nurses did not learn these facts until their liberation from Japanese internment camps in February 1945. Before that liberation they would endure twenty-seven days of the Battle of Corregidor and more than three and a half years in enemy prisons.

Nurses from Bataan soon realized that the tunnel itself could be an enemy. From the moment they walked through the main entrance of Malinta Tunnel, they were attacked by the stench of sweat, blood, unwashed bodies, dirty clothes, overused and undercleaned latrines, and gas gangrene. The odors hung in the still, hot, dusty air like a blanket pressing on them from all directions. One of the first things they noticed was the soldiers sleeping along each side of the tunnel on ammunition cases, on cots, or on the cold, damp cement floor. Ambulances passed within inches of their heads, the bombs that fell day and night shook the rock walls and ceiling from the main entrance to the farthest lateral, and still they did not wake, deep in the sleep that only complete exhaustion can bring. In contrast to the sleeping troops, soldiers assigned to the tunnel rushed about repairing electric lights, sewage drains, and the ventilation system.

Nurses who had worked in the hospital on Corregidor and in the Malinta Tunnel since December led the veterans of Bataan to the nurses' lateral, where they would sleep two in a bed until men assigned to the quartermaster could install additional beds two and three tiers high. The new arrivals were given little time to rest before being added to the work schedule in the hospital laterals.

For an entire week after the surrender of Bataan, Gen. Jonathan

Wainwright ordered that none of Corregidor's large guns could fire on the peninsula for fear of hitting American and Filipino troops left behind. The surrender of Bataan gave the Japanese new points from which to fire their more than 150 artillery batteries at Corregidor. The unmerciful rain of shells began almost immediately and increased in frequency and intensity with each of the twenty-seven days of the Battle of Corregidor. Adding to the devastation of their firepower, the Japanese moved their mortars from Cavite to the hills surrounding Mariveles. With the aid of captured maps, an observation balloon company that floated two Japanese soldiers above the Rock, and information most likely obtained from captured Allied troops by torture, Japanese shells fell with deadly accuracy on Corregidor's gun batteries, its power plant, its water supply, along the east coast beaches exploding Allied land mines, and at the entrances of the Malinta Tunnel. After Corregidor's antiaircraft artillery and gun batteries were destroyed, Japanese bombers, flew lower each day. As April moved into its teens and twenties, Japan reaffirmed its total control of the air over Corregidor.

The depth and solid rock of Malinta Tunnel offered physical safety from bombs and shells but exacted a terrible price from those who sought its refuge. Malinta had never been intended for the numbers of people who would live and work in its damp, dusty confines. The ventilation consisted of three air shafts that ran from the main tunnel and two laterals to the topside plateau, forcing air downward. The air vents had been designed to provide air to underground storage rooms and were woefully inadequate for serving the two to five thousand people who shared the tunnel at various times. To make matters worse, the dry season combined with enemy bombardments added a heavy concentration of dust to the hot air, making breathing a challenge for nurses, doctors, staff, and troops and almost impossible for the patients. Lt. Helen Cassiani described those conditions: "Dirty. Dusty. Hot. We had no air conditioning, of course. And we even had to wear masks—wet masks in order to breathe," she said. "We would take gauze and wet it, put it over the patients' mouths in order for them to breathe a little bit more comfortably. When the shelling and bombing would occur, it was even worse because the dust, the little stones would just fall down through the cracks and cover everything."[3]

Between air raids, off-duty nurses, staff, ambulatory patients, and patients in wheelchairs would gather at one of the entrances for what the defenders called "sun snatching." In the evenings, when battle conditions permitted, people gathered at an entrance to listen to guitar music and sing along. On those hot April nights, the air was filled with the voices of patients and nurses signing softly, "To you sweetheart, aloha, from the bottom of my heart."[4]

Food and water continued to be a problem on the Rock. Food was limited to what had been stored in the tunnel months and even years before the beginning of the war. As the Battle of Corregidor wore on, the bakery and water supply were hit numerous times. After one attack, the water supply was knocked out for four days, leaving the troops and medical personnel two choices of beverage: fruit juice or boiled salt water. The fruit juice was served to patients, while everyone else drank salt water flavored with coffee. The problem was alleviated somewhat when the quartermaster, after drilling for two days, finally hit an artesian well.[5]

With each day, the intensity and frequency of the Japanese bombardment increased. Ambulances brought the wounded directly to the hospital lateral where nurses sorted the casualties and stretcher-bearers carried them to surgery or the appropriate ward. The wounded included men with arms, legs, and faces shot to pieces or shot away entirely. Blood dripped from the stretchers as the men were carried into the hospital, staining the cement floor in front of the hospital lateral dark red.

There were no special wards for seriously injured and dying patients. The best that nurses could offer was to screen off certain beds, but privacy inside the tunnel was all but impossible. People were crowded together day and night. The nurses' lateral had one shower, one toilet, and one sink for eighty-five nurses. Frequently, civilian women related to President Manuel Quezon or on his staff would ask to use the nurses' shower. The chief nurse of Corregidor, Lt. Ann Mealer, decided that the women could use these facilities only when they were not being used by the military nurses. Since sanitation was of prime importance in the tunnel, Mealer had to go to the lateral used by the women on Quezon's staff and tell them they were not to empty bedpans used as chamber pots in the sink which they and the nurses used to wash their faces.

Army nurses resented the fact that Quezon's staff were the only civilians in the tunnel who did no work on the upkeep of the tunnel or the care of the wounded. Other civilian women were assigned regular duties by the chief nurse. Young women were trained to take temperatures and fill patients' water pitchers. Older women were trained to roll bandages and make dressings.[6]

A physical ailment directly related to the heat, dampness, and humidity of the tunnel was known as Guam blisters. Most of the nurses contracted them and suffered from the painful skin eruptions and sores they left when they burst. Nurses who had this skin condition on their arms and around their waists found it very painful to move or lift patients but continued with their duties in spite of discomfort.

The nurses were determined to stay as healthy as possible. Lt. Madeline Ullom decided to use a can of foot powder she found in the nurses' lateral to help prevent athlete's foot. "I gave my feet a nice dose of this powder," she said. "The foot powder was too strong . . . and I got an awful infection in my toes." The infection was so bad that doctors decided to do surgery. "They did [an] incision and drainage," Ullom reported. "I had a bandage on my foot for a few days and everybody teased me and said that I just better get well quick or Tojo would come in and he'd catch me. So [eventually] Tojo [the Japanese premier] did come and catch me."[7]

Living in the tunnel also produced emotional stress. The heat and crowded conditions, lack of food, lack of sanitary conditions, lack of sleep because of the almost constant bombardment, and the realization that help was not coming and death or capture was inevitable combined to cause depression and irritability. Added to these conditions was the stress of knowing that although you were alive at 0900, you might well be dead before 1000. Shell-shocked patients were admitted to the hospital with growing frequency. For months everyone on the Rock had been pushed to the edge of human endurance. Now with the enemy's relentless shelling, individual minds were shattering, and brave young men were brought incoherent and trembling to the tunnel. Along with mangled bodies, medical personnel were confronted with broken minds.

Nurses were the primary caregivers for these bloodless casualties of war. Young women only two or three years older than most of these patients, young women who had lived through and cared for the wounded of Clark Field, Fort Stotsenberg, Manila, and Bataan, who knew the same starvation diet, the same heat and dust of battle, the same malaria, dengue fever, and dysentery, the same horror of seeing the torn and twisted bodies of friends, would now care for the invisible wounds of war that would bleed long after all physical wounds were healed. Nurses listened to the stories of horrific events that had exploded minds and now threatened to cast their indelible images forever into the future. One such story was related by Lt. Juanita Redmond: "The boy had been standing at a battery gun talking to a friend. There was shelling going on around them though they seemed to be out of the direct line of fire. Our patient dropped something and bent down to retrieve it, going on with his conversation. As he straightened up, the shell-torn head of his friend flew past his face and the shattered body fell at his feet."[8] Nurses who had not seen psychiatric patients since their days in training learned to care for an increasing number of shell-shocked victims.

One might ask why military nurses who shared the combat zones and cared for its casualties did not experience immediately incapacitating psychiatric problems themselves, especially when their everyday lives were filled with the horrific casualties of war. Weren't women supposed to be kept out of combat areas because they were the "weaker sex" and "could not possibly deal with the tragedies of war"? How, then, were these nurses able to care for men whose minds had been shattered by the same bombing, artillery fire, devastation, and death they too had shared? Unfortunately, these women were not included in studies conducted by the Veterans Administration or Armed Services involving the defenders of Bataan and Corregidor or prisoners of war held by Japan. After interviewing and corresponding with these nurses, reading everything we could find written by or about them, and spending more than a decade investigating and considering the subject, we offer the opinions we have formed and the conclusions we have reached.

We suggest that men and women drawn to medicine, nursing, and the helping professions approach life differently from average citizens and ordinary soldiers. Military men and women in these professions have very different roles from combat troops, and these nurses have more in common in their outlook and training with these men than with average citizens of their own gender. In this sense, medicine, nursing, and helping professions are great levelers for those who feel "called" to their practice. This sense of mission was so pronounced in the 1930s and 1940s that, to use the words of author Frank Slaughter, the call to the healing arts was a "magnificent obsession."

Each of the military nurses in the Philippines and on Guam when World War II started had lived through the Great Depression and had acquired a special discipline and determination characteristic of their generation. They had voluntarily entered a profession that the majority of citizens at the time considered replete with menial tasks, such as emptying bedpans and working with naked bodies and bodily functions. Even as students, their senses were assaulted with sights, sounds, and odors not discussed in polite company. Knowing they would face such sights and despite discouragement from families and friends, these women determinedly followed their calling to help heal. Three years of training to earn the title "registered nurse" would put them close to the struggle and carnage of life and the reality of death. Day by day and patient by patient they would learn the professional attitude that would allow them to help the grievously injured and suffering and to comfort the dying.

As graduate nurses, and again against the admonitions of friends and families, they volunteered for the even more "unladylike" profession of military nurse. Unlike the combat soldiers, whose role value changed drastically once a wound or illness kept them out of battle, the mission of medical personnel was enhanced as combat grew more fierce and casualties increased.

Perhaps the most outstanding difference between the ability of combat soldiers and medical personnel to withstand the horrors of war has its origins in the nature of their training. As many combat veterans have pointed out, no amount of training can adequately prepare a soldier for the horrors of combat. No matter how lifelike the simulated combat conditions, they are still simulated. On the contrary, doctors and nurses train and work with real casualties and life hangs in the balance even while they are learning. The carnage of life—shooting and stabbing victims, burn cases, casualties of car crashes and train wrecks—are an ordinary part of life at a city hospital. Lt. Frances Nash spoke not only for herself but for her colleagues when she said: "Anything the ambulances could pick up still living was brought to us. So what I was about to face and do [care for the casualties of war] in the jungle, I owe to my knowledge from Grady [Hospital in Atlanta] and the hard times."[9] Without their realizing it and without didactic design, their "basic training" had prepared them for the tragedies of war and the combat zones.

Adaptation and improvisation were key skills for nurses on the Rock. One young nurse, five-foot-two-inch-tall Lt. Madeline Ullom remembered that one of her last classes before graduation was on improvising. Ullom, who had decided that she would either remain at Jefferson Hospital in Philadelphia or enlist in the Army Nurse Corps, saw little point to the subject of improvisation. She reasoned that Jefferson Hospital had everything that would ever be needed, and so did the army. She decided there was no need for her to pay attention in the class. Her mind was changed by the kindness of her instructor.

"Doctor Thad Montgomery was the instructor. He had been so nice the first time I ever gave sutures for a major operation. . . . So I decided to pay attention to him when he told us what to do and how to improvise. When our sterilizer went out [in Malinta Tunnel] . . . I remembered he had told us that if you don't have anything [a sterilizer], the best thing you can do is to wrap your materials in two packs and two covers and put them in the oven. If you don't have clocks . . . you keep them in there . . . until the outsides get all brown and singed."[10]

Improvisation was also necessary with clothes. When nurses were evacuated from Bataan, they were allowed to take only what they could carry in their hands. Many now found it necessary to scrounge for clothing. They borrowed from nurses who had not been on Bataan, and some used clothes they found when all men but the wounded and medical doctors were evacuated from the tunnel after the surrender of Corregidor on 6 May 1942.

One of the nurses, Lt. Minnie Breese, found a barracks bag outside the nurses' lateral. "I opened it . . . and it belonged to Colonel Howard Brightong. I knew him. He was a classmate of Stubbs from West Point. I knew his wife and kids too. So I said, I'll just take these. He had all his jockey shorts. They're comfortable for underwear. So I took all his jockey shorts, and he had a small foot. So I had his shoes. Those were my Sunday shoes. I guarded those with my life. He had pants, and all white shirts. . . . I can sew by hand. So I made shirts. Cut the sleeves off, cut them down to fit me and with my skirts . . . they looked nice. I used his underwear, pajamas, and everything else he had in there."[11]

The lack of water became more of a problem as the Battle of Corregidor slipped toward its inevitable end. Salt water was rationed in the tunnel and was used not only for coffee but for showers and all personal needs. Bathing with salt water was a unique experience. Instead of removing dirt and perspiration, the salt formed a layer of its own and caked over the skin, trapping sweat and grime beneath a white, flaky crust.

One of the many things the defenders ran out of on Corregidor was salt tablets. In the humid heat of Malinta, people perspired profusely. Nurses reported that sweat would roll down their legs and collect in their shoes until it sloshed over the sides and made a squishy sound as they walked. Perspiration also complicated the simple act of seeing. Occupants of the tunnel constantly had to wipe away the perspiration that rolled down their faces in ever increasing streams.

It is little wonder that when any break in the bombing and shelling occurred, patients and medical personnel escaped through the tunnel entrances to catch a few breaths of fresh air. "Fresh air" was a relative term, because the air on Corregidor reeked with the odor of gasoline and cordite. Still, compared to the almost unbreathable air in Malinta, even the fresh air of the Rock was an improvement.

At dusk on 24 April 1942, a large group of wounded men were gathered outside the western entrance of Malinta. Patients sat in wheelchairs, lay on pallets on the ground, walked or stood on crutches, or simply sat. Many of the patients were sharing cigarettes, conversation, and a lighthearted mood until a 240–millimeter mortar shell fell a short distance from them. Immediately men started for the tunnel entrance, haltingly on crutches and in wheelchairs, wounded helping wounded as their eyes scanned the skies. Nurses and corpsmen who had heard the scream of the falling shell rushed toward the tunnel entrance to aid their patients.

Heavy iron gates had been installed at each entrance to the tunnel, and the concussion of the exploding shell had slammed the gates shut so they could not be opened from the outside. Nurses could hear pounding on the gates as they approached the entrance to the tunnel from inside. Men's voices were calling for the gates to be opened. When nurses were within five feet of the gates, a second shell exploded in the midst of the wounded, and the air was filled with screams of pain and agony. Nurses and corpsmen swung the gates open and rushed to treat the new casualties.

They met a scene of carnage. The explosion had killed fifteen patients instantly and had severely rewounded more than one hundred. Fifty of those would die before morning. Seasoned nurses who had worked in major emergency rooms in civilian life and had treated thousands of wounded on Bataan went from patient to patient, triaging and treating, with tears running down their cheeks. Every nurse knows the agony of bending over a patient, powerless to help, while the patient dies. The nurses of Bataan and Corregidor were confronted with suffering and death on an almost unimaginable scale. Such experiences reach deep inside the human soul, splitting it asunder and leaving the individual forever changed.

That night patients were carried to the hospital laterals in what seemed an unending line. Sometimes the dead were brought in on stretchers. The nurses who had been working for almost twenty hours told the corpsmen to be more careful and to bring only the living. The exhausted corpsmen replied that they were doing the best they could while working in total darkness.

Everybody was doing the best they could, but circumstances were outdistancing them. In late April, doctors were so overwhelmed that they turned minor surgery over to the nurses. Nurses were performing amputations, removing shrapnel, and suturing wounds. In the wards of the hospital laterals, nurses were treating patients, in beds stacked three tiers high, without the benefit of ladders to help reach them. Nurses had to climb on the foot rails of beds to care for patients on the top level.

The stacking of hospital beds presented special problems when the entire company of a gun battery ate contaminated canned beef and two hundred soldiers were hospitalized with food poisoning. The added load of two hundred patients with severe stomach upset and diarrhea exhausted the supply of emesis basins and bedpans, and nurses improvised with buckets and any size pot or pan they could press into service. The heat and poor ventilation in the tunnel, combined with the vomiting and diarrhea of the patients, filled the hospital and its closest laterals with a sickening and overpowering odor.

By 25 April General Wainwright decided to get as many officers who had been requested by General MacArthur and nurses off the island and safely to Australia, which lay approximately 1,350 miles away. Wainwright asked that two navy PBYs fly from Australia via Mindanao to Corregidor and take out a group of twenty nurses and more than thirty army officers. Given the addition of the twenty nurses and the need for an extra plane, the first response from MacArthur's headquarters was that gasoline was at a premium and could not be wasted on a mission that had little chance of success. Wainwright insisted, and the planes were dispatched with crews that volunteered for the "suicide" mission.

When the U.S. Army Command in Melbourne, Australia, issued a request for volunteers, Lt. Cmdr. Edgar T. Neale, USN, formerly stationed in the Philippines, was designated to lead the evacuation flight. He held a meeting with four pilots who also were familiar with the Philippine Islands. "'We have orders to perform a secret flight and want volunteers,' Neale said. 'You do volunteer, don't you?' We did," Navy Lt.(jg) Thomas Pollock reported.[12]

At 1000 on 27 April 1942 the pilots of the two PBYs, Pollock and Lt.(jg) L.C. Deede, and their respective five-man crews took off from Perth, Australia, on an eighteen-hundred-mile flight. They arrived at 0530 in Darwin, which the Japanese were bombing heavily every day. Neale contacted the army in the Philippines to see if Americans still held their Mindanao landing site and return fuel supply and to set up secret signals for landing on Mindanao. The pilots and crews tried to get some sleep but were continuously awakened by droves of huge flies in the humid 105–degree temperature and the drifting of their seaplanes that were blown about by shifting winds despite the planes' anchors. They had to restart the engines frequently and reanchor to keep the planes from colliding with the brush along the riverbank. At 1500 they expected to take on the usual thousand pounds of cargo. Instead, three thousand pounds of medicine, radio repair parts, and antiaircraft nose fuses were loaded, all bound for Corregidor. The PBYs were so crowded that the crew had to crawl on their hands and knees to get through the plane. At 1630 they departed from Darwin. They were undertaking a 1,350–mile journey over enemy-held territory, with navigation charts that did not show all of the islands or their proper shapes. For twelve hours they flew north through rain squalls and heavy clouds with no stars for celestial navigation, hoping to avoid detection by the Japanese, whose aircraft operated from the islands below, and finally arrived on Mindanao.[13]

At 0730 on 29 April, Emperor Hirohito's birthday, the Japanese began a punishing five-hour bombardment of the Rock. Lights in the tunnel went out for several hours. In the operating room, doctors and nurses operated by flashlights until a small emergency generator was placed into service. Lt. Hattie Brantley remembered the blackness of those hours: "If you ever want to feel what the darkness of Egypt was like, you should be in a tunnel, in a cave, when the lights go off. You can feel it, and sometimes this [the lights] would be off for hours."[14]

Toward noon, General Wainwright received word that two PBYs had reached Mindanao and would be on their way to Corregidor that night. Wainwright and Capt. Kenneth Hoeffel, senior naval officer on the Rock, selected the water between Caballo Island and Corregidor as the safest place to land the planes. Wainwright delegated the selection of the fifty evacuees to Colonel W.E. Cooper, his chief surgeon; the chief nurse, Capt. Maude Davison; and several other officers.

General MacArthur earlier had requested that Col. Stewart Wood, Wainwright's assistant chief of staff, and several cryptographers, whom he named, be among the fifty evacuees. Colonel Cooper named nine officers, brigadier generals, colonels, lieutenant colonels, and two civilian women to be included in the group.

Capt. Maude Davison, the five-foot-two-inch-tall, fifty-six-year-old chief nurse of the Philippines and veteran of World War I, gave two of her senior nurses the choice of whether to go or stay. Both nurses, Lts. Ann Mealer and Josephine Nesbit, declined places on the planes and chose to stay with their patients.

At 1800 that evening Captain Davison ordered twenty nurses to report to the mess hall. She told them that they were relieved of their duty assignments on Corregidor and would leave that night on navy flying boats for Australia. She went on to instruct the twenty women that they were not to speak of their planned departure, nor were they to say good-bye to anyone.

Nurses selected to leave were torn between the desire to return to the United States alive and the duty they felt toward the patients. Two of the nurses asked Captain Davison if they could give their places to a specific individual. They were told they could not. They were under direct orders as officers in the Army Nurse Corps, and they had no choice but to obey.

Even though none of the twenty evacuees had said a word to anyone about leaving, several nurses and medical personnel were at the tunnel entrance to wish the departing nurses good luck. General Wainwright escorted the nurses to the docks and helped them board a small boat that would take them to the waiting planes. Ten of the nurses climbed aboard the first plane, along with fifteen other evacuees; the other ten boarded the second plane with fourteen other evacuees. At 2345 both planes took off and headed for Mindanao where they were to land and refuel on Lake Lanao.

Before the second plane could reach the lake the following morning, it ran into heavy fog and had to land on Lake Tarac for approximately thirty minutes, waiting for the fog to lift. When the fog dissipated, the PBY took off and landed shortly on Lake Lanao, where the twenty nurses were reunited.

The Japanese had landed on Mindanao that morning and were only about forty miles away from the two planes. Although General MacArthur's headquarters had instructed the crews that they were to pick up several more passengers at the Del Monte Plantation airfield, the evacuees headed first for the closest army installation by bus. The military encampment near the lake provided the planes' passengers with a breakfast of hot cakes, coffee, bananas, and coconuts. Later, en route to the Del Monte Plantation airfield to pick up additional passengers, the Americans encountered the Japanese. Several times along the road, they jumped from the bus and took cover in rice paddies when Japanese planes swept down over their path and strafed them.

The group reached the airfield safely and were served a second breakfast of fresh eggs and strong coffee made with fresh water. Some of the officers were reunited with old friends from Manila. They shared several bottles of champagne and drank to the "good old days" and to the future. Meanwhile, the planes' crews were securing their aircraft.

At 1500, when the passengers returned to their planes, the pilots directed them to get rid of most of their belongings to accommodate the weight of the passengers who were being added. Nurses and most officers threw away their canteens. The majority of air corps officers abandoned their pistols and holsters to lighten the load.

Boats arrived and carried ten nurses and others to the first plane. The PBY taxied several times but failed twice to take off. Just as the nurses on board feared they were not going to get off Mindanao, the third takeoff attempt succeeded, and the plane lumbered into the air, gained altitude, circled several times, then headed toward Australia. The nurses who were watching from the second plane felt confident that the next morning they would be reunited with their comrades. Unfortunately, they were wrong.

The second plane, piloted by Lt.(jg) Pollock, hit a reef as it maneuvered into position for takeoff. "About that time there was a rending sound as the hull struck a submerged coral reef," Pollock said. "Water came pouring in. Some of the passengers put blankets over the holes and stood on them. I started the motors as the plane pivoted into the wind and started to taxi. Word came forward that we were taking water fast and not try to take off."[15]

The passengers were sent to the Del Monte Plantation while the crew attempted to repair the damaged plane. By then the plantation had its own problems, not the least of which was being cut off from its water supply. Nurses and their companions brushed their teeth with pineapple juice and ate lavishly of the only food available—fresh pineapple.

The plane's crew, aided by several navy and army air corps men, worked on the plane continuously. When Comdr. F.J. Bridget returned from the Del Monte Plantation, he was surprised to find the plane still afloat. Pollock told the commander that he still had hope that he would be able to fly the plane out. Bridget informed Pollock that the army was sending a B-17 from Australia to pick up the party and that if the seaplane was not functional by then, Pollock and his crew could ride out on the B-17.[16]

Hours later, the PBY was repaired enough to attempt a takeoff.

There was no guarantee it would fly, but believing a B-17 was on its way to Mindanao to pick up his previous passengers, Pollock decided to give it a try. With several thousand pounds of water in its hull, the PBY, along with its original crew, climbed laboriously into the air and made its way toward Australia.

For the next forty-eight hours, the stranded Americans moved from one airfield to another in hopes that the promised B-17 would arrive before the advancing enemy troops reached them. By the time they entered the town of Impalutau, the consensus was that they could no longer depend on being rescued. They decided to split up. The men would try to locate an American-Filipino guerrilla unit in the hills, and the nurses would remain at a small civilian hospital, renamed Force General by the military. The hospital was operated by an American missionary doctor who had spent more than twenty years in Japan before opening the hospital on Mindanao. Shortly after the attack on the Philippines, the doctor was commissioned as an army officer. The group hoped that the physician's background and the fact that he spoke fluent Japanese would prove an asset to the nurses when dealing with the Japanese military.

Around 1 May General Wainwright learned that the U.S. submarine *Spearfish* was returning to Australia to be resupplied with torpedoes. Wainwright requested that the submarine stop in Manila Bay and take ten military nurses, one navy officer's wife, and fourteen army and navy officers to Australia with them.

The only nurse General Wainwright named to leave on the submarine was Lt. Ann Mealer, chief nurse in Malinta Tunnel. Colonel Cooper, Wainwright's chief surgeon, told Mealer that she was approved to leave Corregidor that night. When Cooper reported to Wainwright, he told him that Ann Mealer had declined the opportunity to leave the besieged Rock. General Wainwright was sincerely touched by Mealer's decision: "Colonel Cooper came to me . . . and reported that Lieutenant Mieler [Mealer] had told him she did not want to leave ' . . . as long as there's a patient in the hospital.'

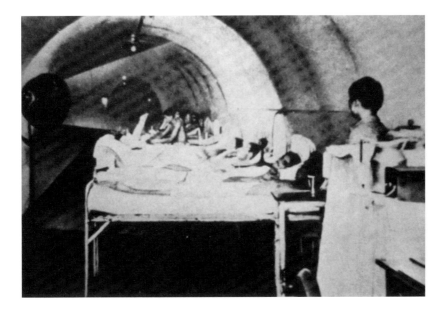

Wounded troops in hospital lateral in Malinta Tunnel on Corregidor, 1942;
U.S. Army Signal Corps.

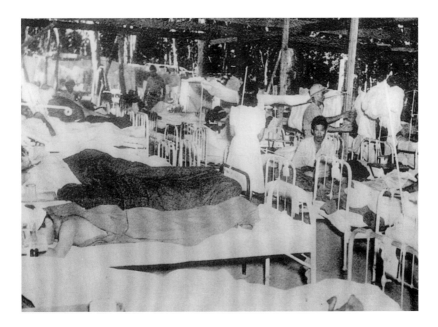

Gas gangrene cases in field hospital on Bataan; U.S. Army Signal Corps.

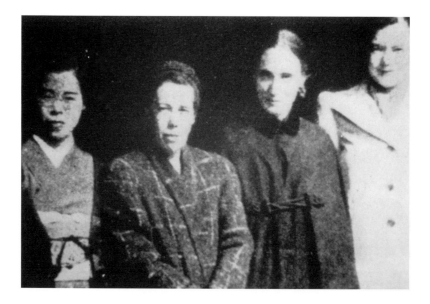

Japanese woman and three of the five POW navy nurses captured on Guam and taken to Japan in January 1942; Japanese Army photo.

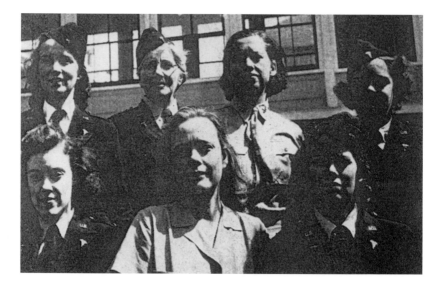

Members of the Army Nurse Corps who were successfully evacuated from Corregidor by PBY in April 1942. (Left to right): Juanita Redmond, Florence MacDonald, Ressa Jenkins, Harriet G. Lee, Dorothea Daley, Mary Lohr, Eunice Hatchitt; U.S. Army Signal Corps.

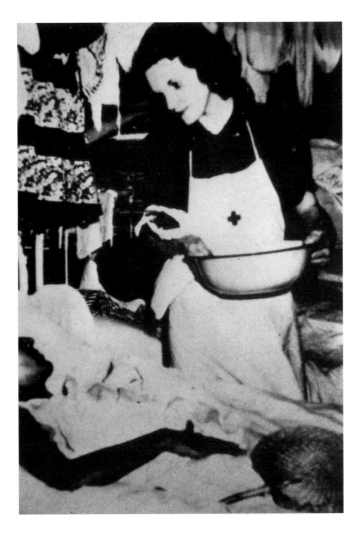

POW navy nurse Margaret Nash caring for a civilian internee
in the hospital at Santo Tomas; photograph taken by a
Japanese soldier.

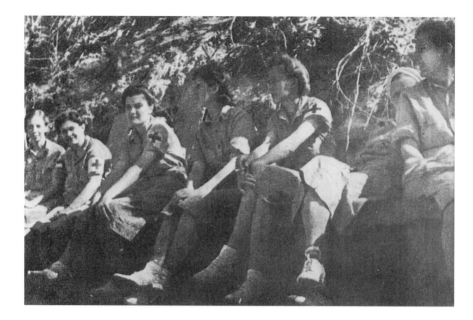

Army nurse POWs lined up at entrance to Malinta Tunnel for Japanese 14th Army propaganda photo hours after Corregidor was surrendered. Left to right: Vivian Weissblatt, Adele Forman, Imogene Kennedy, Beulah Greenwalt, Eunice Young, Eleanor Garen; Japanese Army photo.

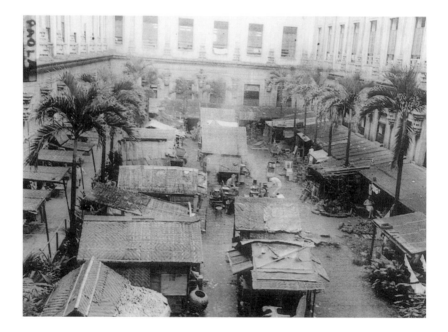

Shanties built by internees in the courtyard of main building, Santo Tomas Internment Camp; U.S. Army Signal Corps.

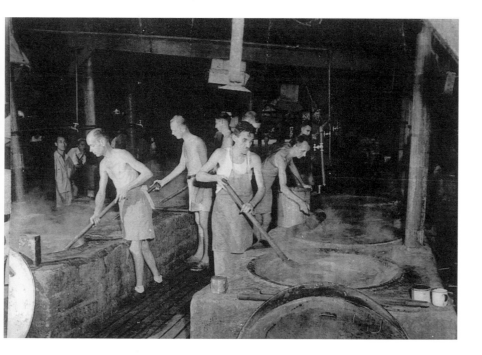

Civilian internees used large vats to cook the little food available at Santo Tomas; U.S. Army Signal Corps.

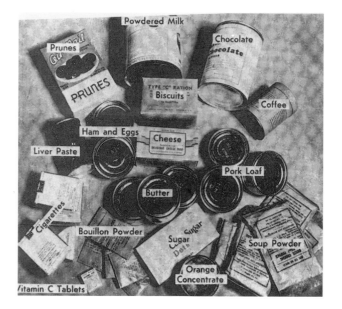

Contents of comfort kit sent by Red Cross to POWs and civilian internees in the Far East. POW military nurses received two such kits during their more than three-year internment; American Red Cross.

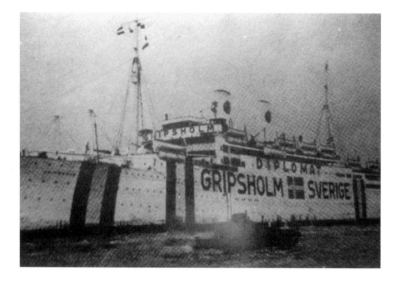

Red Cross ship *Gripsholm* carried comfort kits meant for POWs and internees and acted as transport in a prisoner of war exchange in the Far East during World War II; American Red Cross.

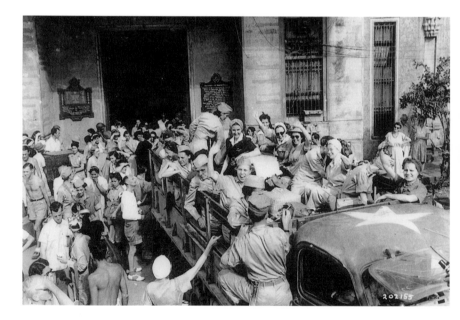

U.S. Army nurses recently freed at Santo Tomas climb into trucks that will carry them to a waiting plane on Dewey Boulevard; U.S. Army Signal Corps.

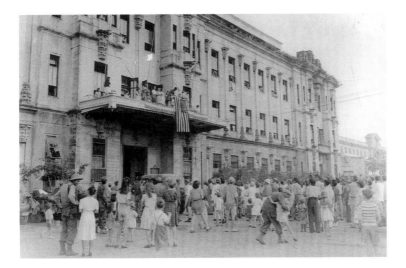

First display of the American flag following liberation of Santo Tomas, February 1945; U.S. Army Signal Corps.

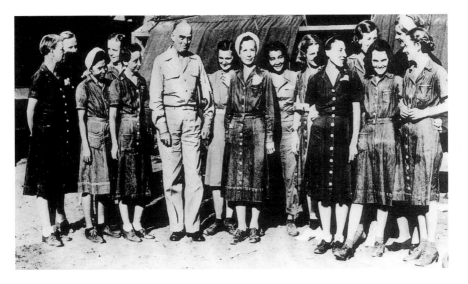

Navy nurses are greeted by Vice Admiral Thomas C. Kincaid, USN Commander 7th Fleet and Southwest Pacific Force, after their liberation from Los Baños Internment Camp on 23 February 1945. (Left to right): Lt. Susie Pitcher; Lt. Dorothy Still; Mrs. Basilia Stewart, a naval officer's wife who worked with the nurses in the prison camp hospital; Lt. Goldia O'Haver; Lt. Eldena Paige; Vice Adm. Kincaid; Lt. Mary Chapman; Lt. Comdr. Laura M. Cobb, chief nurse; Miss Maureen Davis, a civilian nurse who worked with the navy nurses; Lt. Mary Rose Harrington; Lt. Helen Gorzelanski; Lt. Bertha Evans; Lt. Margaret Nash; Miss Helen Grant, a British nurse who worked with them; and Lt. Edwina Todd; U.S. Navy photograph.

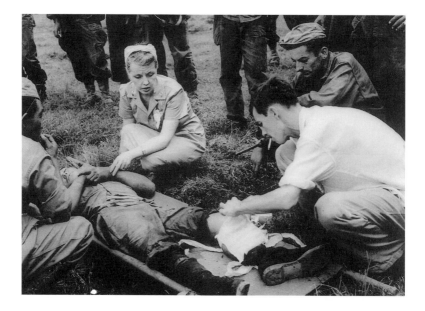

U.S. Army nurse 2d Lt. Frankie Lewey, administering medical treatment to a wounded Japanese soldier following the liberation of Santo Tomas; U.S. Army Signal Corps.

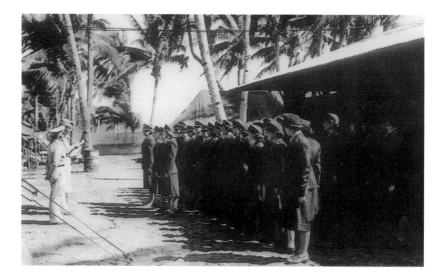

On 20 February 1945, Brig. Gen. Denit, chief surgeon, SWPA, awarded the Bronze Star and promotion to the former POW army nurses at Telesa, Leyte Island, before their departure for the U.S.; U.S. Army Signal Corps.

I considered this a truly great act of heroism. She knew as well as I that she was signing her captivity warrant."[17]

The USS *Spearfish* received twenty-five evacuees from Corregidor on 3 May 1942. The evacuees—eleven army nurses, one navy nurse, one navy wife, six army officers, and six navy officers—were taken by small boats to rendezvous with the submarine, which lay approximately four miles southwest of the Rock. Once they had slipped silently through the hatch, they saw how limited the space was. For the first twenty-two hours of the trip the *Spearfish* submerged and evacuees were told to talk and move around as little as possible. The instruction was hardly necessary, because conditions were so crowded on board that several people passed out from the lack of oxygen combined with the starvation diet they had lived with on Bataan and Corregidor. To help combat the problems created by overcrowding, extra oxygen was pumped into the ventilation system and lime was spread about to cleanse the air.[18]

The spirits of the escapees were lifted by the many kindnesses of the submarine's crew, who showed unbounded willingness to help them in any way. "The submariners were so good to us; they gave us some of their clothing since we had lost everything we owned," Lt. Lucy Jopling said. "In particular I remember the cut-off dungarees, which I had never seen before, and T-shirts."Something else about the submarine trip that Lucy Jopling would never forget was the instructions for flushing the commode:

There were three heads (commodes) in the submarine and we [nurses] were assigned one. The instructions to flush it were to be adhered to implicitly or the powerful shower that would come flying up out of the commode was unimaginable! These instructions went something like this: Before using, see that bowl flapper valve "A" is closed, see that gate valve "C" in discharge pipe line is open, and that valve "D" in water supply is open. Then open valve "E" next to bowl to admit necessary water, close valve "D" and "E." After using, pull lever "A." Release lever "A." Open valve "G" in air supply line. Rock air valve "F" lever outboard to change measuring tank to 10 pounds above sea pressure. Open valve "B" and rock air valve lever inboard to blow overboard. Close valve "B," "O" and "G." So the Filipino mess boy nearby did it all for us. It was embarrassing.[19]

On 20 May 1942 the *Spearfish* disembarked its passengers and cargo safely at Fremantle, Australia. Included in the cargo were all the nurses' pay records so meticulously cared for by Lt. Josephine Nesbit on Corregidor.[20]

On 4 May the Japanese shelling of Corregidor reached its zenith. Between 0700 and 1200, 1.8 million pounds of Japanese artillery shells fell on Corregidor. The torrent was so overwhelming that General Wainwright and General George F. Moore used mathematical calculations to figure the rate and number of shells that fell during that five-hour period. They concluded that Japanese gun batteries hit the Rock with a five-hundred-pound 240–millimeter shell every five seconds between 0700 and 1200. This meant that twelve shells fell every minute, a total of thirty-six hundred in five hours—enough shells to fill six hundred army trucks.[21]

On that same horrible day, Corregidor withstood thirteen air raids. It was evident to everyone on the island that this punishing bombardment was a preinvasion tactic. The Japanese military would attempt a landing in a matter of hours. What would it mean for the first American military women to experience combat conditions for almost five solid months and then be taken prisoners of war? The knowledge of the atrocities perpetrated by Japanese troops on the women of Nanking hung heavily over Malinta. When the Japanese troops arrived, would they respect the nurses as military officers? Would they be allowed to remain with their patients to care for American and Filipino sick and wounded? Or would they be molested, raped, and killed? In the end they decided that they would have to carry on with their work as long as possible. "We had discussed the possibility of rape and it was just one of those things," Lieutenant Brantley said. "We kept taking care of our patients. We stayed on the wards at the bedside . . . we kept doing what nursing care we could."[22]

The shelling and bombing were so intense that the sounds of explosions never stopped. The concussions shook the ground beneath their feet and cracked the rock over their heads. The number of men brought to the hospital suffering from shell-shock increased dramatically on 4 and 5 May. A lateral that led to the hospital was opened as a psychiatric ward and three-tier bunks were installed for the patients. Lt. Phyllis Arnold was placed in charge and instructed to put these soldiers to bed, give them water, and cover each with a blanket.[23]

Nurses were told to remain dressed at all times and to wear the Red Cross armbands they had been issued when the Battle of Corregidor began. Colonel Theodore T. Teague, who had been a prisoner of war in World War I and had been a member of General MacArthur's staff, gave advice to the nurses concerning what they might expect when the Japanese came into the tunnel.

The nurses gleaned as much as they could from Colonel Teague's talk and applied it as best they could to their own situations. Lt. Anna Williams related some of her preparations: "I expected they [Japanese] would take anything they wanted of ours, that was jewelry or anything that we had with us of that sort. I had a wrist watch, that I used for taking care of patients and then I had a little gold one that was a dress watch . . . I also had a couple of rings," Williams said. "I made a rat [a hairpiece] and put it in my hair with the good watch and the rings and brushed my hair back over it. So I carried those out of internment with me. . . . The one [watch] that I used for taking care of patients, I plastered it all with sticky tape so that I just could see the second hand. To keep a pen was a big thing because they took all the fountain pens they saw around the place, but they never did take my watch because it looked so beat up."[24]

One nurse, Lt. Verna Hively, a twenty-seven-year-old from Long Beach, California, was asked by a wounded soldier to take his West

Point ring home with her when she went and to give it to his wife and daughter. She gave the officer her promise, and more than three years later she kept it.[25]

At 2330 on the night of 5 May, Japanese troops landed men, tanks, and flamethrowers at the eastern end of the island. Around the same time, a Japanese shell hit the west entrance of Malinta Tunnel and closed it off completely. Two entrances remained open—the main east entrance and the northern entrance which led directly to the hospital laterals.

The night of the invasion, officers who had not been outside Malinta to fight since landing on Corregidor came to the nurses to say good-bye. They wore helmets and carried gas masks and guns. Lt. Ann Mealer remembered her last night in Malinta Tunnel before the surrender: "The firing just went on all night long and casualties were brought in all night long. Sometimes the shelling would be so hard the compression of the shells would blow your skirt tight around your legs in the operating room."[26]

Time was growing short for the defenders of the Rock. The last message that went from Corregidor to the outside world was as follows:

> They are not near yet. We are waiting for God knows
> what. How about a chocolate soda. (Pause) Not many.
> Not near yet. Lots of heavy fighting going on. (Pause)
>   We've only got about one hour 20 minutes before. . . .
> (Pause)
>   We may have to give up by noon, we don't know yet.
> They are throwing men and shells at us and we may not
> be able to stand it. They have been shelling us faster than
> you can count. . . . (Pause)
>   We've got about 55 minutes and I feel sick at my
> stomach. I am really low down. They are around now
> smashing rifles. They bring in the wounded every minute.
> We will be waiting for you guys to help. This is the only
> thing I guess that can be done. General Wainwright is a
> right guy and we are willing to go on for him, but shells

were dropping all night, faster than hell. Damage terrific. Too much for guys to take. Enemy heavy cross shelling and bombing. They have got us all around and from the skies. (Pause)

From here it looks like firing ceased on both sides. Men here all feeling bad, because of terrific strain of the siege. Corregidor used to be a nice place. But it's haunted now. Withstood a terrific pounding. (Pause)

Just made broadcast to Manila to arrange meeting for surrender. Talk made by General Beebe. I can't say much. Can't think at all. I can hardly think. Say, I have 60 pesos you can have for this week-end. The jig is up. Everyone is bawling like a baby. (Pause) They are piling dead and wounded in our tunnel. Arms weak from pounding key long hours, no rest, short rations, tired. . . . (Pause)

I know now how a mouse feels. Caught in a trap waiting for guys to come along finish it up. Got a treat. Can of pineapple. Opening it with signal corps knife. (Pause)

My name Irving Strobling. Get this to my mother, Mrs. Minnie Strobling, 605 Barbey Street, Brooklyn, N.Y. They are to get along O.K. Get in touch with them as soon as possible. Message. My love to Pa, Joe, Sue, Mac, Garry, Joy and Paul. Also to my family and friends. God bless 'em all, hope they be there when I come home. Tell Joe wherever he is to give 'em hell for us. My love to you all. God bless and keep you. Love. Sign my name and tell mother how you heard from me. (Pause)

Stand by.[27]

Finally, word came over the tunnel radio that General Wainwright would surrender Corregidor effective at 1200 on 6 May 1942. The announcement came as a relief to troops and medical personnel who had been pushed beyond human endurance. Nurses hated the idea of surrender but were glad it would mean an end to the creation of new casualties.

In the psychiatric ward shell-shocked soldiers had had the opportunity to sleep for many hours in Malinta's relative safety. The rest and news that they would not have to return to unmerciful bombing and shelling in unprotected topside positions had a positive effect on almost all psychiatric patients. "Then we learned that Wainwright had gone to surrender," Lieutenant Arnold said, "what I did was, when it calmed down in the afternoon, I went up and down the aisle and whispered in their ears, 'We've surrendered, go back to your unit.' And sure enough they got up and walked out."[28] There are no records and no way of knowing for certain the severity of the psychiatric breaks these men had suffered. At the end of World War II, however, psychiatric cases in the southwest theater stood at 43.94 per 1,000 of the average strength per year, the highest of any theater of operations. Dealing with the tropical climate and jungle, combined with the brutality, unpredictability, and fanaticism of the Japanese military, presented greater stressors for American soldiers than in any other war zone. The second highest incidence was experienced in the Mediterranean theater.[29]

After the white flag was raised, the Japanese continued to shell Corregidor about every fifteen minutes. They told General Wainwright that they would not accept the surrender of the Rock unless he also surrendered all Allied troops in the Philippines. As an added incentive to Wainwright, the Japanese threatened to use flamethrowers inside Malinta and its laterals. Realizing that the annihilation of the American and Filipino troops on Corregidor would not add one jot to the strength of other Allied troops in the islands, Wainwright finally agreed to the Japanese conditions of surrender.

With the Japanese acceptance, the bombardment of Corregidor was at last stilled. Hundreds of wounded who could not make it to Malinta during the barrage presented themselves at the hospital for treatment. Nurses triaged and administered morphine to patients waiting for surgery. In the midst of newly arrived casualties, the Japanese military entered Malinta Tunnel and the hospital laterals.

Nurses had been told by Chief Nurse Maude Davison to continue their duties as far as was practicable and not to go off alone at any time. How nurses experienced the arrival of the Japanese troops depended largely on where they were when the enemy entered the tunnel. Lt. Ann Mealer, who was acting as part of a surgical team, got her first glimpse of the enemy when Japanese troops entered the operating room. "I was giving an anesthetic to a case that had been shot through the leg, and they were putting a plaster cast on him at that point. They'd already finished the surgery," Mealer said. "I thought they'd be officers. Instead they were just like you see these old Japanese field soldiers with caps with tails. . . . The flap goes down the back over their necks and they asked me in perfect English if that table was sterile. I said it has been but they're putting plaster on now and I said it's not sterile anymore." Mealer felt her heart pound against her chest as they walked over to the instrument cabinet and looked into it. "We had a set of instruments that somebody had taken off a dead Jap soldier in Bataan. . . . They were cleaned up and sterilized and put in that cabinet and I thought sure they'd recognize it but they didn't."[30]

Japanese officers walked through the tunnel and hospital laterals inspecting conditions and asking questions about the patients. Japanese doctors questioned army medical officers and nurses concerning the diagnoses and conditions of many of the patients.

Lt. Hattie R. Brantley was somewhat relieved when the tunnel was not overrun by hordes of Japanese soldiers. She recalled that the hospital area was placed off-limits to the majority of Japanese soldiers and that the soldiers and officers who came into the tunnel spoke English. In fact, several of the doctors had been educated in the United States and spoke excellent English. Brantley was in charge of the orthopedic ward and remembered that the Japanese took the time to be sure that each person in traction was there for medical reasons and not hiding out from the imperial army.[31]

Lt. Madeline Ullom remembered that about two hours after the Japanese entered the tunnel, Capt. Maude Davison gathered ten nurses and told them that the Japanese wanted them outside the tunnel for a picture. The nurses were lined up with the commanding officer and the chief nurse. A Japanese soldier with a rifle and bayonet stood guard at each end of the line. "A Japanese officer who spoke excellent English said, 'We are going to take your picture and we're going to send it to General MacArthur to show that you are alive and that we are looking after you. Don't be afraid. I know how you Americans feel. . . . I'm a graduate of one of your universities.'"[32]

As a stipulation of the surrender agreement, General Wainwright insisted that the nurses would not be molested by any member of the Japanese military or anyone under their control. General Homma and his staff reluctantly agreed but added their own stipulation—no nurse would have any contact or conversation with any Allied soldiers or officers. Nurses were permitted to speak with medical officers only when discussing patients or receiving orders for their treatment.

In the first forty-eight hours after their arrival, groups of Japanese officers toured the nurses' quarters at all hours of the day and night. On the first attempted foray by high-ranking Japanese officers into the nurses' lateral, the party had no sooner drawn back the sheet covering the doorway when they were met by Capt. Maude C. Davison, drawn to her full five-foot-two-inch height, right palm raised, shouting, "Halt! You cannot come in here until my nurses are dressed." Without a word the group waited for ten minutes until Captain Davison reappeared, lifted the sheet, and bade them "Come in."[33]

After that nurses slept in their duty clothes. A nurse was posted as a guard to ring a bedside bell when Japanese military came to the lateral on what seemed "sight-seeing tours" to the nurses, and all the women would stand at attention beside their beds until the Japanese left. After several days of broken sleep for all the nurses, Captain Davison went to her commanding officer and complained vigorously about the practice. That afternoon two signs were posted in Japanese stating that the hospital area and the nurses' quarters were off-limits to everyone except the Japanese high command. The signs joined others sprinkled liberally throughout the tunnel stating in Japanese that all equipment in the tunnel was the property of the imperial Japanese government.

In the first two days, the Japanese cut off all ventilation to the tunnel. Temperature, humidity, and odors rose to almost unbearable levels. An announcement that nurses and medical personnel would be allowed to go to the entrance of the tunnel for thirty minutes each day was greeted with relief. That relief lasted until the first trip individuals made to breathe in fresh air. "One day, it must have been three or four days after [the surrender]," Lieutenant Ullom said, "I was out at the edge of the door [entrance] of the tunnel. The bodies were lying all around on the ground. Of course, by that time they were all swollen up terrifically. Oh, it was awful. The sights were just horrid. . . . They were Americans. I remember one was a marine. He was an officer. A major."[34]

American military commanders repeatedly asked the Japanese for permission to bury their dead, but it was not granted for almost a week. Finally, the Japanese allowed the dead to be cremated, but without any religious ceremony. Once the dead were cremated, the Japanese allowed nurses and medical personnel to walk outside the tunnel entrance for approximately one hour a day. While walking, no one was allowed to speak. The practice lasted for about ten days.

During the first week after the surrender, all able-bodied men not essential to the operation of the hospital were removed from the tunnel. At the same time, doctors were ordered to discharge patients as soon as they were able to return to duty. The pressure for discharge continued until many patients not ready to leave the hospital had to be released as fit for duty.

In mid-May a Japanese soldier was brought to the Malinta operating room, suffering from acute appendicitis. A Japanese doctor performed the surgery with an American surgeon acting as his assistant. The medical team was appalled when the Japanese doctor wanted to insert a drain and leave the inflamed appendix in. "No, you don't do that," the American surgeon said. "The appendix had better come out, and you give him sulfa." The Japanese doctor followed the advice.[35]

The patient was placed in a bed in a hospital lateral, and a Japanese soldier was stationed beside him day and night. Apparently the Japanese were afraid the man might be poisoned or harmed by

American medical personnel. Ironically, it was the soldier guard who raised the ire of an army nurse. One day while Lieutenant Mealer was walking down the hospital lateral she saw the Japanese guard, wearing only a G-string, walking toward her. "And I thought, my heavens, what a disgusting sight. So there was one of the doctors that spoke Japanese, and I said, 'Would you please tell that Japanese to go and get his pants on.'" Mealer got a piece of khaki, gave it to the doctor, and said, "If he doesn't have any [pants], tell him to have some made." With a little reflection, she added, "Now that I think of it, if he'd shown up in that khaki, I guess his commanding officer would have killed him. I don't know what he ever used that khaki for, but he never came down that tunnel any more in that outfit."[36]

In approximately three weeks, the nurses were moved out of their regular lateral into another section of the tunnel. Their new quarters had triple-tier bunk beds and every bed was filled with its own complement of bedbugs. Captain Davison took the bunk closest to the lateral entrance where she could keep an eye on anyone approaching.

The new lateral came with an unexpected advantage—it was connected to the bathroom that had been used by General MacArthur, and through a hole in the bathroom wall, the nurses could see what they suspected was one of the navy storage areas. They remembered that the navy had stored a large amount of canned food and flour in their lateral. All the nurses agreed it would be worth the risk to enter the lateral because they might find food they could use to supplement the sparse rations given to them by the Japanese.

Lt. Minnie Breese recalled one of the trips to the navy storage area. "We'd wait for the guards to go by at the other end and we'd holler, and she [Lt. Josephine Nesbit] got in there and she raised up too quickly and smashed her head—but we got all this flour. Big ration cans," Breese said. The nurses hid the cans in their foot lockers and hoped that if and when they were moved, they would be able to take the flour with them.[37]

One mystery that remains unsolved unfolded approximately

four days after Corregidor was surrendered. The Japanese appointed several American enlisted men to accompany them as they followed a very detailed map of Malinta Tunnel in search of supplies placed in the laterals years earlier. Using the map as a guide, the Japanese told the men where to break through lateral walls, which proved to be thin plaster in these areas. On the other side of the designated spots, the Japanese found sacks of cornmeal with Red Cross markings and field kitchen-sized cans of meat, fruit, and vegetables. There were many large sealed tins of fresh water and an entire field hospital, including tents, quinine, sulfa, sutures, and dressings. All of the supplies were carried out of the tunnel, placed on a Japanese ship, and taken away to benefit Japanese troops. It has never been adequately explained how the Japanese knew of the location of these supplies and the Americans did not.

On 24 June the Japanese announced that nurses and patients who could be moved would be transferred the following morning to the old hospital at Topside. Early the next day, all ambulatory patients and the nurses walked and climbed to the bombed-out hospital. More seriously ill patients were left in the tunnel in the care of corpsmen and a few doctors. Since the rainy season was in progress, patients who were able helped build a partial covering for the bomb-damaged wards.

Nurses were delighted to find gardenia bushes in bloom nearby, and they picked the blossoms for each patient's bedside. After six weeks of imprisonment in the tunnel, fresh air, even with rain, and the sweet fragrance of flowers, seemed like a small piece of heaven.

Many of the nurses had or developed dengue fever, malaria, and dysentery while at Topside. Unless completely incapacitated by their illnesses, they remained on duty, taking care of their patients.

Nurses were devastated at having to leave seriously ill patients in the tunnel. They were forbidden by the Japanese to reenter the hospital lateral for any reason. Lt. Ann Mealer had been taking care of an artillery officer whose pelvis had been fractured when the large gun he commanded backfired. She wondered daily how her former patient was faring without the aid of a registered nurse. "So

I went down there one time after I was sure there [weren't] any Japanese guards [around]. We had a badly wounded man. He'd been in the hospital for months. He was in bad shape, and I went down to see him. His name was Captain White . . . and he did not have a mosquito net over him. Lord, he wouldn't sleep a wink because the mosquitoes were huge and it was the rainy season," Mealer said. "So I went out in the yard and chopped some wood for poles to attach to the bed. They had a place for it, for rods . . . and [I] put a mosquito net over him . . . he said, 'I'm afraid that you people will eventually desert me because I'm . . . no good for anything.' I said, 'They won't desert you. They'll take you right along with them'— and we did."[38]

On 2 July the Japanese placed the patients and all medical personnel except the nurses on a freighter anchored offshore. All the men were placed in the hold of the ship and kept there without water or food. On 3 July all but twelve nurses were marched to the dock. These twelve, including Lts. Madeline Ullom and Ann Mealer, were too ill to walk the distance and were taken to the dock by truck. The nurses were placed on a small boat and taken to the freighter three hundred yards offshore. They were then ordered to climb aboard the ship, each carrying the small suitcase she was permitted to take. Lt. Madeline Ullom remembered that climb: "I had a temperature of about 104 degrees that day. We had to climb up a rope ladder on the outside . . . with that elevated temperature, I did pretty good until I got about three rungs from the top. Everything started going around. I knew that the bay was full of sharks and if I fell in the water, that was the end of it. So I did two more rungs and got up."[39]

As the ship sailed toward Manila, a Japanese officer served the nurses tea and rice cakes on the deck. In perfect English, he told them that they were being taken to Manila, on the outskirts of the city, where a hospital had been set up and equipped in a school. He said as soon as they got to Manila, the men would be unloaded first and brought to the hospital. The nurses would follow and take care of them there.

It was the best news the nurses had received in weeks, and as the ship sailed for Manila, they had a new feeling of relief. "At least," they thought, "we can care for our own sick and wounded casualties." Unfortunately, time would prove them wrong. To paraphrase Sir Winston Churchill, it was not the end of their time in hell, it was not even the beginning of the end; it was, in fact, the end of the beginning.

7

The City of Hell

When we are winning, we can afford to be generous. . . .
Commandant A. Kodaki, Santo Tomas Internment Camp, 1942

When the Japanese ship carrying the wounded soldiers and the army nurses arrived in Manila, the nurses were assured again that the wounded would be taken to a hospital on the outskirts of the city where they could care for them. The hospital, they were told, was set up in a schoolhouse and was already equipped with beds and medicines. The anxious nurses felt relieved as they watched their patients being off-loaded and placed into trucks that carried them in the direction of Paranaque, where their captors said the school was located.

Finally, the army nurses were disembarked and placed on board two open trucks, each carrying several Japanese guards armed with rifles with fixed bayonets. The trucks started away from the harbor, supposedly toward the hospital where the wounded Americans would be waiting. Suddenly, Madeline Ullom realized that they were not headed for Paranaque at all and decided they needed help finding the way. "I thought they were probably lost, and I knew the way, so I could help them. I told them they were on the wrong road, and pointed toward the right one," she said. "They didn't respond so I told the guards again. 'This is not the right road. The road to Paranaque is the next road up.' The next thing I knew, they tapped me on the back with a bayonet. I decided they didn't want my help, and that I'd best keep quiet."[1]

The trucks did not stop until they reached Santo Tomas University, which had been converted into Santo Tomas Internment Camp in January. As they pulled through the gates and stopped, the nurses were greeted by hundreds of men and women who were anxious to receive word of their relatives and friends who had been on Bataan and Corregidor. Internees were everywhere, standing on the lawn, on the steps, and leaning out of windows, calling and waving at the new arrivals. No contact between the army nurses and the internees was permitted.

When the Japanese ordered the army nurses to get off the trucks, they refused. They told their captors that they were military nurses and wanted to be taken to a military camp so they could care for their wounded. The Japanese insisted, flashing their bayonets and pointing their rifles at the disobedient nurses. As Lt. Hattie R. Brantley put it, "When someone with a bayonet insists you get off the truck—you get off."[2]

The women were hurried into a room where they were fed a mixture of rice, fresh pineapple, and shreds of carabao meat. It was the first fresh fruit that they had eaten in months. After this meal, the Japanese searched them and their meager belongings (what one musette bag could hold) and questioned each about her past, including her life in America. When the interrogations were completed, the inquisitors reloaded the women onto the trucks and transported them across the street to Santa Catalina girls' dormitory. Both Santa Catalina and Santo Tomas were surrounded by a high fence which was interworked with sawali, a thatched pattern of palm leaves, making it impossible for anyone to see in or out of either institution.

The fifty-eight POWs were placed in an upstairs room, where, except for their two meals a day which were taken in a room downstairs, they would remain for six weeks. The rest of the lower level was occupied by nuns who had worked at Santa Catalina before the war. Meals were brought over from Santo Tomas in large containers and placed on a table in the downstairs room. When the internees carrying the kettles had left, the nurses were permitted to go downstairs to eat. The empty containers were picked up later after the women had returned to their crowded living quarters upstairs.

Sleeping facilities consisted of a native version of a lounge chair. The bamboo frame was curved and the backing of the chair/bed was provided by thatched cane that sagged as if it had seen many nights of hard use before its current occupants arrived. The native beds were placed so close together that there was barely an inch between them.

During this time, their only contact with the rest of the camp was through the Japanese guards and a minister who was permitted, at their request, to conduct Sunday services twice. "I guess the Japs thought of it as a silent debriefing period," Lieutenant Brantley said. "They wanted us to forget all the horror and atrocities we'd seen, and not mention them to the internees in the camp."[3]

The six weeks at Santa Catalina, with no work assignments, stood in stark contrast to the strenuous activities, hectic pace, and emotional turmoil of the last six months on Bataan and Corregidor. The absence of bombing and strafing, after months in the heart of a combat zone, and the relatively good food, compared with what they had eaten since December 1941, allowed the nurses to rest and regain some of the strength and energy they had spent caring for the thousands of wounded, ill, and dying, and living the minute-to-minute life of soldiers in the thick of war. At the end of the six weeks, a Japanese officer told the group that they would be placed with the other internees in Santo Tomas, but the nurses were not to speak of anything that happened on Bataan or Corregidor.

When the army nurses were released into the general population of Santo Tomas on 24 August 1942, the camp held 3,290 internees in extremely crowded conditions. Of these internees, 2,339 were Americans and 875 British, of whom 2,045 were males. Like internees who had entered before them, each nurse was issued an enameled plate, a metal cup, and a spoon that would serve them until their liberation in 1945. Meals and other activities of daily life had become established before the arrival of the American army nurses. On 1 July, after tireless efforts by the Executive Committee, a group of businessmen who were elected to represent the internees, Japanese authorities accepted the responsibility for feeding the camp's population. Before this date, their captors had denied any responsibility for providing food for "civilian internees who were not covered under the rules for treatment of Prisoners of War." Santo Tomas had depended on the Philippine Red Cross (American Red Cross) for food from 4 January until 11 July. From the first of July, the Japanese allocated seventy centavos daily for each internee, and from this total, the Executive Committee paid for all utilities, construction, maintenance, sanitation, and medical supplies. Approximately forty-eight centavos per capita were committed to food (approximately U.S. twenty-four cents).

The food at Santo Tomas for the first year and a half was adequate but by no means plentiful. The central kitchen served two meals a day, which were essentially identical. Internees stood in a long chow line twice a day to receive a scoop of lugaw, a cornmeal mush, a ladle of very watery rice called moogow, and a dipper of mostly vegetable water with a few vegetables and small pieces of meat.

People with money were able to buy food to supplement their rations. The Japanese ran a camp store that sold fruits, vegetables, cigarettes, and other foodstuffs. In addition, Filipino vendors were permitted into camp to sell food items such as fruit, vegetables, eggs, and sugar. Prices were high but nothing compared to what they would become as the years wore on and food became less and less available.

Unlike many wealthy civilians, army nurses had arrived in the internment camp with few possessions and no money. They had been warned on Bataan and Corregidor to destroy any money and checks in their possession, and they followed instructions to the letter. Now they found themselves in a situation where money could allow them to buy the food supplements that would change their barely adequate rations to a more nutritious diet. They would need to borrow money and, fortunately, a secret loan process had been arranged by several of the men on the Executive Committee, including Carroll C. Grinnell, Chief Executive Officer of General Electric in the Far East, and Earl Carroll, Chief Executive Officer of Insular Insurance in the Far East. Others who also made money available were executives with Coca-Cola, Pennzoil, and other American companies. These business executives used the credit of their corporations with Chinese and Swiss banks to bring money in surreptitiously. Doing anything surreptitiously was no easy task given the approximately fifty Japanese soldiers who guarded the camp and the many informers among the internees. Despite the constant danger, army nurses borrowed for themselves, and Capt. Maude C. Davison borrowed money through Grinnell for some of her nurses. These women signed small pieces of paper promising to repay the money when the war ended. Most nurses borrowed $100 to $150 at a time, and by the time they were liberated, many owed about $1,000. As conditions in the camp worsened year after year, borrowed money could mean the difference between life and death.

Lt. Rita Palmer remembered signing IOUs while a prisoner of war. "I think most of the nurses borrowed money. The business-men thought we were a good risk because we would get our pay when we got home, and they would get their money back," she said. "We signed little chits, we'd borrow so much. Then when we got home, General Electric sent me 'You owe us this amount of money.' I paid what I owed. And then General Electric sent me the slips I had signed at Santo Tomas."[4]

For the moment, food was not a major problem and no one was in immediate danger of real hunger, let alone starvation. In time, the nurses and internees would know firsthand what both felt like and what they could do to the human body and spirit.

Army nurses were first assigned to live in the mining building. The Executive Committee assigned some of them the job of clean-ing the women's latrines. Since the nurses were certain they could be of more help doing the jobs for which they were trained, Capt. Maude C. Davison, chief of army nurses, visited the Japanese com-mandant and explained that her group were military nurses and should be assigned to a prisoner of war camp where they could care for their own wounded and ill soldiers. After the comman-dant made it clear that this was not an option, Davison insisted that the army nurses be assigned to the hospital and clinic to care for the internees. Maude Davison, a seasoned army nurse, was not easily put off or frightened and was determined that her nurses would be treated with dignity and be allowed to practice their profession. The army nurses were reassigned to establish a hospital in Santa Catalina dormitory and take over the nursing care in the clinics and hospital wards of the camp; several nurses were assigned to work outside of camp in civilian hospitals.

The hospital set up in Santo Tomas involved various camp buildings. The Santa Catalina school building housed a men's and women's ward on the second floor and a clinic on the main level. A communicable disease hospital was established in the mine building for the many internees suffering from tuberculosis, and a separate children's hospital served the camp's six hundred inmates under age sixteen. Clinics were operated in the main building, the education building, and the gymnasium.[5]

The army nurses were moved to the second floor of the main building, where their quarters consisted of four rooms that had previously been classrooms. The rooms were directly opposite the Japanese guardhouse. Each nurse was allocated a bed space of six feet by three feet, with a one-foot aisle between each bed. Personal belongings were kept on and under the bed, the only space in the camp that one could consider her own. This "ownership" allowed the illusion of personal space but did not protect against Japanese searches. Lt. Anna Williams mentioned several ways the nurses tried to improve their living space. Some got boxes and built shelves that fitted over the foot of the bed. To reduce the risk of colds, they slept head to toe.[6]

With living space, food, and work assignments taken care of, the army nurses settled into the daily routine of the camp. On the day shift, nurses worked four hours a day, because of the heat and humidity. Nurses on the night shift worked eight to twelve hours. Shifts were shared equally until several nurses, including Eunice Young and Earlyn Black, volunteered for permanent night duty.

The day in Santo Tomas began for the general population at 0600, when a record was played over the loudspeaker. Nurses who were on the morning shift got up about 0515 to get a head start on the usually crowded bathroom facilities. The second floor of the main building housed three hundred women and had three showers, five washbasins, and five toilets to serve the entire floor. Privacy was a thing of the past, a luxury that disappeared when the Japanese attacked the Philippines. Madeline Ullom recalled: "Somebody, usually Peggy O'Neill, would wake us up early so we could get a shower before the rest of the floor was up and headed for the bathroom. At other times, there would be six or seven people under each shower, trying to get a sprinkle."[7] Some especially modest women showered with their underwear on. In the second floor women's bathroom, someone had posted a hand-printed sign that read: "If you want privacy, close your eyes!"

One of the only places a person could find any semblance of privacy was the main toilet area on each floor. Each stall had a cotton curtain in front of it and was the safest place to read any notes that were smuggled in or thrown over the camp wall.[8]

Like everything else, clothes were very scarce in camp. Army nurses wore khaki skirts and shirts as a duty uniform. They were glad to have colorful shirts, given to them by civilian internees, to wear off duty.[9]

Everyone in camp over the age of sixteen was designated to do a camp job. Some of the older internees were assigned to "tissue issue," distributing toilet paper to internees. Men were issued two sheets a day, and women were allowed four. The Japanese-controlled English newspaper that came into the camp daily was a blessing. Once read, it was quickly divided for bathroom service in a society where paper was as scarce as hens' teeth from the first day Santo Tomas opened its gates.[10]

Two things that were plentiful in camp were flies and bedbugs. As early as February 1942, the Sanitation Committee issued fly swatters and organized a "Swat-That-Fly Campaign." A junior "Swat-That-Fly" club was organized for children, and the three youngsters who killed the most flies were awarded prizes. The children joined the campaign enthusiastically and shared in the feeling of doing something to benefit the entire camp.

To combat the vermin that would easily have taken over the camp, the Sanitation and Health Committees designated special weekly campaigns such as "Clean Mosquito Net" week and put up posters to remind internees that constant vigilance was needed to prevent the spread of vermin that could bring sickness, disease, and death. One poster, "They Crawl by Night," listed the "confessions" of a bedbug, along with a cartoon drawing of the culprit. Military nurses did all they could to attack and eliminate the pests. They carried their bamboo beds outside and poured boiling water into them. When the beds were back in their dormitory, they placed the legs of each in a small can of water, hoping that the nonswimming vermin would no longer be able to crawl onboard.[11]

During off duty hours, internees could avail themselves of more than forty-six courses offered by professors and professionals who had taught or practiced in Manila before the war. The students had to take the courses without benefit of textbooks, paper, or pens. Japanese soldiers had long ago claimed fountain pens and wristwatches as souvenirs so classes were conducted without the assistance of either. Nurses took courses in such subjects as Spanish, philosophy, history, and astrology. There were also lessons in bridge and chess, and clubs for each met regularly once or twice a week.

During the afternoon hours, many people observed a siesta time, while others did their laundry behind the main building. Internees had constructed a long concrete stand with several basins built into it, and people would stand in line to wait their turn to do their washing. "When you washed your clothing, you went out and laid it on the grass," Lieutenant Brantley recalled. "There were no such things as clotheslines. You laid it on the grass and sat by while it dried because somebody could steal it if you looked the other way."[12]

Food was important to every internee. A noon meal was provided for teenagers, internees over eighty years of age, internees who worked at least four hours a day, those with a doctor's certificate, and those who worked preparing vegetables for camp meals.

Between noon and dinner, internees frequently visited the Filipino vendors who were allowed into the camp to sell fruit and other foodstuffs. Their purchases were often added to their evening meal to improve its nutritional value. Everyone had a bucket and would line up at chowtime and make their way to the food service station, where a ladle of rice with vegetables or a few rare shreds of unidentifiable meat was placed in each bucket. Ration in hand, the nurses would return to a wide corridor in the main building where "families" had separate tables and added whatever extras they had managed to collect and shared the evening meal.

As time passed and food was no longer available from vendors, the nurses were dependent on what the Japanese provided—largely rice and totally inadequate. But for a time, extra food could be purchased by those with the money to buy. Eggs could be bought for about five cents each, bread for less than fifteen cents a loaf, and fruit such as an orange or a banana for approximately five cents apiece.

After the evening meal, internees would carry their lawn chairs outside to sit in groups to talk and listen to recorded music played over the loudspeaker from 1700 to 2100. Donations of phonograph record collections from civilians who had lived in Manila before they were interned provided Santo Tomas with thousands of records and a wide variety of music from which to choose each evening. One evening would be dedicated to big band music, another to western music, another to classical music, and so on through the collection.

Confinement created its own brand of boredom necessitating a variety of projects and special events for internees. The camp was also fortunate to have a huge library of books brought into Santo Tomas from universities and private collections. Reading was a favorite pastime for the nurses, and books were one of the preferred living quarters for the bedbugs. Despite the presence of these unwelcome pests, nurses took advantage of the time to read widely from the classics and books as current as *Gone with the Wind*.

One navy nurse recognized the need for reading material to aid in her survival. Lt. Edwina Todd had not been well since she and the other navy nurses at Santa Scholastica had been moved to Santo Tomas in March 1942. The camp doctor informed Todd that she would not live to return to the United States. "I thanked him, but I was mystified why he ever bothered to tell me," she said. "I couldn't make a will . . . there was no one to tell." What Todd did was stop her nursing duties and establish the Anchor Library for POWs. The library consisted of books and magazines the prisoners had with them when they were captured. "I knew my survival depended on getting a little more to eat . . . and if you had some money you could buy it," Todd said. "Books were rented out at 5 [cents] a day and 25 [cents] a week. (People who didn't have any money could trade reading material.)" There were several other navy nurses in the project with Todd. The nurses made the glue for the book tags from sour mash and used whatever scraps of paper were available. For identification they drew a blue anchor on each library card and book.[13]

Internees on the Entertainment Committee acquired a piano and provided stage shows mixed with music and comedy skits. As time went on, the stage that began as several boards nailed to wooden crates in the west patio of the main building was moved to the front of the main building next to the movie screen and rebuilt more sturdily. The new location inspired the name, Little Theater Under the Stars.

During the rainy season, broadcasts of "talk shows" and plays were presented over the loudspeaker system. This allowed internees to remain indoors out of the rain and still have entertainment that helped raise their morale.

On 9 September 1942 the nurses from one of the PBYs that left Corregidor in May were brought to Santo Tomas and imprisoned with the other army and navy nurses. They had been taken prisoners of war on 10 May 1942 but stayed at Force General until 17 August, when they and 110 civilians were moved to Davao, a POW camp. "The trip was made by truck and in the hold of an indescribably verminous freighter. Many of the civilians and nurses were ill from recurrent malaria and fatigue," Lt. Alice Hahn, a twenty-four-year-old nurse from Chicago, Illinois, said. The army nurses and a mixed group of civilians were held in a Catholic convent at Davao, Mindanao. It was there that the nurses tasted their first fresh fruit in many months. A week passed before the captives were told that they were to be repatriated and were placed on a freighter for Manila. After waiting on the ship for several days, the party was brought to Santo Tomas.

At Santo Tomas on 29 September the Japanese authorities made a surprise inspection on the package line and shed. They searched all outgoing packages for notes and found more than fifty. The notes were confiscated, and the package line was closed indefinitely. The internees, who depended on the package line for food from outside, were now obliged to stand in the camp's chow line for their meals. This increase in the number of internees being fed caused delays in meal service and put a strain on food supplies. A sawali fence was installed at the gate to cut off contact between package bearers and recipients, and the package line reopened in early October.

As a further step in exercising their authority over the internees, the Japanese ordered that all flashlights in camp be turned over to them as of 23 October. After the flashlights were confiscated, thefts inside the camp increased, and the Executive Committee increased the number of internee "police" patrolling the camp. As conditions in Manila worsened, many of the thefts were committed by people who scaled the wall to steal from internees.

By mid-November, the Executive Committee was faced with spiraling prices for the food it purchased for the camp. The price of sugar had increased 100 percent, coffee, 10 percent, and beef from 5 to 10 percent. On 16 November the internees' ration of sugar dropped from four tablespoons at breakfast to three.

During the third week of November, there were so many rats in camp that they constituted a menace to health. The Sanitation Committee initiated a special effort to reduce the rodent population by assigning some of the internees to seek and destroy the pests and to place poisons in various locations. One subcommittee would revisit the poisoned sites to dispose of the rodent cadavers.

On Thanksgiving Day, 26 November 1942, internees received a turkey dinner and watched the "East-West" football game played by camp teams. They dubbed the game "the Talinum Bowl," for talinum, a green vegetable similar to spinach, which grew with little encouragement in the Philippine Islands.

The camp canteen was expanded on 29 November to sell additional items for internees' use. Basic products such as toothpaste and soap became available.

On 1 December chow-line tickets were issued to internees to cut down on the number of people going through the line more than once or requesting meals for nonexistent people so as to steal food. These internees became known as "food chiselers" and were deeply resented by fellow internees.

A British relief ship arrived with Christmas comfort kits for the internees. The ship also brought relief staples for the camp. These supplies were from the South African Red Cross Society and contained 566 sacks of provisions, packed in individual kits, four kits to the sack; 543 cases of canned meat and vegetables, 48 one-pound cans each; 242 cases of corned beef, 24 eight-ounce cans each; 160 cases of dried fruits, 25 pounds each; 75 cases of cocoa, 14 kilos each; 14 cases of vitamin caramels, 35 kilos each case; and 300 sacks of sugar, 100 pounds each.[15] Because of the limited number of individual kits, the Executive Committee decided to give one kit to every two internees. Each kit contained small cans of meat spread, bacon, condensed milk, margarine, marmalade, pudding, tomatoes, cheese, soda crackers, tea, sugar, a cake of chocolate, and a piece of soap.

Lt. Eunice Young recorded in her prison diary: "December 23, 1942—Comfort kits given out. X-mas entertainment. 1st movie we had seen in a year. Toilet paper rationed 8 sheets per person. Soap 1 bar per week. X-mas party—ice cream and cake with money engineers sent us. [U.S. Army engineers were kept on Corregidor to make changes that the Japanese wanted in the fortifications.]"[16]

On Christmas Day several religious services were held before the internees received a special holiday meal. The army nurses enjoyed turkey and fruit cake sent in to camp by a Mrs. Hube, a naturalized American citizen and former army nurse who was married to a wealthy German businessman in the Philippines. Since Japan and Germany were Axis powers, the Japanese allowed Mrs. Hube many privileges such as supplying the military nurses with extra food. The Christmas entertainment was concluded with a concert given by the combined men's and women's choruses, followed by the internees singing Christmas carols. More than two thousand internees attended the celebration, seated in their lawn chairs on the plaza in front of the main building.

In her book *To the Angels*, Lt. Maude Denson Williams recorded the events of that first Christmas in Santo Tomas. "And it [Christmas] was a good one. Visitors came in, more than 700 of them, to see their relatives and friends, and they came loaded with baskets and boxes. Many families spread their picnics on the ground and sat around feasting. . . . After the visitors left, we gathered around the Christmas tree back of the main building, and watched Santa Claus arrive and deliver almost 2000 wrapped gifts to the 435 children under twelve. [The toys had been handmade by internees over the previous few months.] For once, we seemed like normal people living under normal conditions. The Japanese sent photographers for pictures to use as propaganda. But who cared? They hadn't contributed a thing to our celebration, and we could be sorry for them because they hadn't one of their own."[17]

The day after Christmas, the second relief ship arrived, carrying food from the Canadian Red Cross. The relief supplies delivered were as follows:

36 tins orange juice, 100 imperial oranges each
36 cases jam, 24 two-pound cans each
274 cases provisions in individual kits, 16 to each case
32 cases toilet articles in individual kits, 20 to each case
5 cases cigarettes, 500 packages each
3 cases pipe tobacco, 144 pocket-size tins each
5 cases assorted clothing
1 case shaving cream
1 case powdered milk (klim), 27 five-pound cans
1 case biscuits (cookies), 135 pounds total

4 cases dehydrated potatoes, 2 fifteen-pound cans each

135 pounds soap powder

Each toilet kit contained a safety razor, five blades, a toothbrush, shaving brush, shaving cream, toothpaste, toilet soap, comb, needles, thread, and a thimble.[18]

Internees who went to the docks to unload the relief supplies returned to camp and reported that they had seen many cases of hospital and medical supplies piled up on the piers, marked Squibb and Parke-Davis and each labeled "American Red Cross." When the medical supplies did not show up in Santo Tomas, the Executive Committee wrote a letter to the camp commandant asking what progress was being made in obtaining the medical supplies that had been requested months ago. The commandant informed the committee that no such supplies were available. On 31 December, the *Manila Tribune*, a Japanese-controlled four-page daily circulated in camp as propaganda, carried a story stating that Japanese military authorities were making a gift of scarce medical supplies to the hospitals in Manila. Grinnell, realizing where the Red Cross supplies were headed, wrote a letter to the commandant requesting that the hospitals in Santo Tomas be included among the recipients of the Japanese benevolence. He did not receive an immediate reply.

The Christmas of 1942 was a high point in the more than three years that would be spent in Santo Tomas. With each passing month, hunger would draw closer and closer to the camp, until starvation had touched everyone and claimed the lives of many. The long slide into the heart of hell had begun.

8

Life along the River Styx

*I don't consider myself a hero. None of us do. But even
though women were not supposed to be on the front lines,
on the front lines we were. Women were not supposed to be
interned, either, but it happened to us. People should know
what we endured. People should know what we can endure.*

Lt. Col. Madeline Ullom, USA, NC (Ret.)

The new year brought word from the commandant that a small
quantity of medical supplies had become available and could be
delivered to Santo Tomas for a specified price. The Executive Committee immediately put plans into motion to borrow the money
needed to purchase the supplies that, until the Japanese had confiscated them, were a gift from the American Red Cross.

Medical supplies were always scarce in Santo Tomas. The Japanese provided none when the camp opened. Along with food for
the first six months of the camp's existence, medicines and supplies were left to the devices of the internees and, like food, became
less and less available. When notified of their impending internment, physicians grabbed whatever medicines and equipment they
could and brought them in pillowcases or other sacks to Santo
Tomas.

Lt. Ann Mealer remembered that medical care inside the internment camp was improvised. "We'd take strands of hemp and

roll it around, string it out, wrap it around tongue blades [tongue depressors] and sterilize it for sutures. Skin suture only."[1]

There was a large supply of morphine in camp but no oxygen. For the first year and a half, internees requiring surgery were sent outside to a civilian hospital. When this practice was no longer permitted, nurses and doctors were dependent on what anesthetics and medications were already in camp. There was a supply of ether, sodium pentothal, and various anesthetics for spinals.

On 6 January 1943, comfort kits received the day after Christmas were given to internees. A diary kept by Lt. Eunice Young during her years at Santo Tomas has provided much valuable information concerning life inside the camp. Although she was in constant danger of being caught, this twenty-eight-year-old nurse from Arkport, New York, took the risk and left a priceless record for history. From that diary we know that the comfort kits from the Canadian Red Cross contained small cans and packages of cheese, tea, soup, corned beef, salmon, sardines, jam, crackers, sugar, raisins, prunes, butter, and powdered milk. At this time Young was also enjoying several books, including *Berlin Diary* by William Schirer, *A Thousand Shall Fall* by Hans Hake, and *Keys to the Kingdom* by A.J. Cronin. The good feelings brought by food and books contrasted with the concern engendered by the dengue fever that was ravaging the camp and sending people to the hospital two on a stretcher.[2]

In January the Japanese tightened up regulations. On 20 January, after announcing that the husbands of pregnant women would be punished by spending time in jail, all pregnant women were sent to San Jose Hospital in Manila. Shanties, nipa palm leaf "houses," open on two sides, were now to be used only by couples over fifty years of age and women with children under ten years of age. Fathers were allowed in shanties from 1000 until 1400. In February, as the rules were becoming stricter and prices were going up, Lieutenant Young wrote in her diary: "Will we ever get out of this place? There has been no news in days, and morale is very low."[3]

Spirits rose slightly as rumors of repatriation made their way around the camp. But any good feelings were counterbalanced by hardships such as the shortage of soap, which was expensive if it was available at all. Adding to the bad news, the sugar ration was cut to three tablespoons per individual per day. Two weeks later, the ration was cut to two tablespoons.

Sugar was high on the internees' wish list. Navy nurse Lt. Margaret Nash, a five-foot, one-inch-tall native of Wilkes-Barre, Pennsylvania, decided to take advantage of a Japanese guard's desire for one of her two wristwatches to barter for the sweet stuff. In November 1941 Nash purchased a watch with the intention of sending it to her niece as a gift for her upcoming high school graduation in June. In a 1945 article titled "The Joys of Meeting," Lt. Mary Jane Brown described how Nash got the most for that watch. "Sugar was what they wanted most," Brown said. "This watch caught the eye of a Japanese guard as he patrolled the internees' camp. He stopped and offered Peg two kilos [of sugar] for it. She displayed it tantalizingly and replied, 'No, me want sugar.' The knowledge that he would be shot if he were caught bartering made him hesitant regarding the sugar, but Peg constantly tantalized him with the watch, pointing out its beauty and value. Every time he'd pass, she would remark, 'Nice Elgin watch, twenty jewels.' This constant goading of his desire for the watch brought about the desired result at the end of a week, and he brought the sugar—twelve pounds. Twelve pounds of precious crystals which everyone craved." [4]

During the third week in April, the camp was shown its second movie, *Gulliver's Travels*, but it provided little distraction from the rising prices being charged by food vendors inside the camp. By 29 April 1943, food prices had risen considerably and were still going up. Eggs were selling for fourteen cents each; margarine, ninety cents for one-quarter pound; pineapples, twenty to thirty cents; bananas, three for ten cents; bread, thirty cents a loaf; canned milk, seventy-five cents a case; and vinegar, forty cents a quart. Essential nonfood items were also costly. Soap was five cents a bar; needles, ten cents each; thread, four cents per spool; matches, fifteen cents a package, a spool of cord, twenty-five cents; toothpaste, six to ten cents; and the all-important toothbrushes for $5.30 each. [5]

Clothes were wearing out and replacements were harder and

harder to find. The husband of one of the English women made knitting needles out of bamboo, and most of the nurses learned how to knit. Lt. Hattie Brantley described some of those efforts: "We knit socks and bras and panties out of grocery store twine. . . . I could turn the heel of a sock just as easily as my grandmother could."[6]

The twine was provided to the nurses by Mrs. Hube. Knitting clothing out of twine did not produce the most elegant items, and sometimes the result was garments of an unusual character and limited utility. In her book *To the Angels*, Maude Denson Williams described some of her efforts and results with knitting.

Since I knew nothing about the knitting art, Earleen [Francis] helped me get started by casting on the stitches for a pair of underpants. . . .

At the top—the band of the garment—a small hole was made to provide for a narrow strip of elastic. When the knitting was finished, the display gave us lots of laughs. For one thing, the white pants had black elastic (the only color available) inserted through the holes. For another, the pants were at least eight or ten inches too long; comments were made that the crotch of the pants might be exposed at the hem line of a skirt. Someone remarked that the knees might get tangled up in the over long pants and cause the wearer to trip herself. . . . It was finally decided that the project be unraveled and the underwear shortened several inches. With the yarn [twine] left over, Earleen would teach me to knit ankle socks. . . . I struggled to knit a pair of socks out of the hard twine. . . . I tried to wear the socks, but the rough, stiff twine hurt my feet. "These socks are crippling me," I complained. . . . "Rip them up and split the twine. Then you can knit two pair of socks," said Earleen. . . . Earleen knit a pair of socks for me which I wore. . . . The split twine made the socks soft and pliable. . . [and] I wore [them] on duty as part of the nurse's uniform.[7]

On 9 May 1943 at 1900, the Japanese announced that eight hundred men would be transferred to an internment camp at Los Baños on the fourteenth. Volunteers were solicited for this first phase in the planned eventual move of the entire population of Santo Tomas to Los Baños. This new place of imprisonment was approximately fifty miles southeast of Manila, at the Agricultural College of the University of the Philippines. The college covered sixty acres and had approximately fifteen concrete classroom buildings and five two-story dormitories. In addition, there were thirty or so small cottages that had been built for use by the faculty. Internees from Santo Tomas would exchange an urban setting in Manila for rural surroundings. Dr. Lynch asked the chief nurse, Lt. Laura Cobb, a forty-nine-year-old navy nurse from Wichita, Kansas, with twenty-three years of navy experience, if she and her navy nurses would volunteer to go to Los Baños to care for the men who were being transferred. The navy nurses went willingly. They left for the railroad station by truck and to music played over the camp's loudspeakers. The navy nurses did not know it then, but they had already experienced the best part of the journey. Lt. Cobb recalled the miserable train trip to Los Baños. "We were placed in steel boxcars, 65 to a car (where normally 30 men would have been a load), one to two nurses placed in a box-car with men (we were thought to be held as hostages provided any men tried to escape). There was one Jap guard in each car. Both doors were closed when the train got underway. After some persuasion, the doors were opened. Some of the men were almost suffocated. Upon arrival at Los Baños, we were taken by truck to our new camp. Upon arrival we were herded together. Jap officers made the nurses sit out on the grass with cups in our hands, pretending we were having tea with them, while others snapped pictures of us."[8]

The following day, 15 May 1943, navy nurses began work at the shell of what had been a well-equipped and organized Filipino hospital in the camp. The Japanese had forced the Filipinos to take all their equipment and leave the facility. Lieutenant Cobb described their first day of admitting patients to the camp hospital and recalled that patients had to bring their own beds and sheets. Since they had practically no equipment or medical or surgical supplies, some men in the camp improvised much of what was needed. They constructed beds, tables, and trays from bamboo and wood; cooking utensils; an instrument sterilizer for the clinic; enema cans; urinals; bedpans; and hand and foot basins from corrugated tin taken from roofs.[9]

As a result of a Japanese rule ending the use of shanties at Santo Tomas, buildings and the chow line became miserably crowded with hundreds of people who had spent much of their time in the shanties and had cooked and eaten their meals there. The eating utensils that these people had used were now stacked in every available empty space in already cramped corridors. Finally, even the Japanese tired of the deliberate overcrowding and permitted people to return to the shanties. At this time several shanties were put up for sale and Maude Denson Williams and Edith S. Shacklette purchased one together. Williams described that shanty and its location:

The location was ideal—near the camp garden, and about 100 yards from the main building—which made it convenient for getting our chow and buying produce from the market and canteen. Bamboo poles tied together with strips of bamboo twine made the frame; the roof was of dried palm leaves, and the floor of thin bamboo planks with cracks between, making the shanty cool and easy to clean. The walls were all plaited sawali, and all the windows were fixed to stand open in case we invited male guests to share a meal. We paid 117 pesos [$58.50] for the shanty, and considered it a bargain. . . . The shanties were private places where we could take our ease with a book, where it was quiet and calm, and our possessions were handy and in order. Places for quiet conversations with friends, pretending we weren't at war, we weren't hungry or bored, or uncertain of our future. We could wonder aloud how far our military forces were in their fight to get to us, and discuss the latest scuttlebutt from Tokyo heard on a secret radio and passed on to someone who passed it on to someone who passed it on to us.[10]

On 21 May Lt. Eunice Young wrote in her diary: "My second birthday as a Jap prisoner. Surprise birthday party for me, ice cream and cake. Dinner at Denny's shanty. A much happier birthday than a year ago. Coffee cut to five A.Ms. a week, tea the other two A.Ms. Sugar reduced to one tablespoon per person [per day]."[11]

In May several cases of infantile paralysis were diagnosed in the camp. Medical and nursing personnel were relieved when the cases proved to be isolated and no epidemic ensued. As was true for many illnesses affecting the internees, the best that could be offered was some relief of symptoms and good nursing care.

The rainy season cut down on outdoor entertainment, and internees were glad for "radio shows" broadcast over the camp's loudspeaker system. Food was becoming less and less available even for those who had the money to buy extras. The regular menu in the chow lines left people always hungry. The menu for 1 June was typical: "June 1—Breakfast—1 cup tea substitute, 1 spoon sugar, 1 large ladle corn meal mush. Lunch—1 plate mongo beans cooked with beef. Dinner—1 plate vegetable and beef stew, 1 banana, 1 cup unsweetened tea substitute."[12]

As summer and the rainy season wore on, food continued to be a top priority. On 9 June Lieutenant Young wrote in her journal: "Needed money, so sold my raincoat for 60 pesos. It's the rainy season, but rather be wet than hungry . . . 45 pesos today from Miss Davison. Did have hopes of getting out of here in a few months, but looks now as if it might be years."[13]

In mid-June Japanese authorities announced that every internee would be issued a ration card for clothing. The yearly allowance was eighty points, and the points did not go far—a dress, pants, and one pair of socks took all eighty.

Despite problems with food and clothing, nurses were more than willing to help the American army liberate the Philippines. One opportunity to hasten their liberation presented itself to Lt. Anna Williams, who in 1943 worked the day shift outside the camp at the Philippine General Hospital. She was approached by an undercover guerrilla leader, a Filipina nurse in charge of the cancer clinic, and asked to provide information concerning the size of the guard force at Santo Tomas and where the guards were positioned on and off duty. Williams agreed to help and told Miss Misscean that since all army nurses were being assigned to duty inside the camp, she would have to enlist the help of someone who could get in and out. José Agrilla, a Filipino nurse who worked at Santo Tomas and also worked at the IBM office in Manila, immediately came to her mind. She had been told by Eddie Yarborough, an interned American, that Agrilla was very loyal to America and lived just outside Santa Catalina Hospital with his parents and sisters.

Lieutenant Williams contacted Agrilla through a friend, and he met with her in the hospital room of a Miss Fullertoon, a Scot and former nurse who was one of several very ill patients assigned to Williams's care. The four rooms that housed these "critical care" patients were located along one side of the building and overlooked Agrilla's home and garden. Even though Japanese soldiers were quartered on the first floor of his house, José Agrilla agreed to carry the messages from Williams to Miss Misscean. They planned a signal to indicate there was a message for Agrilla to pick up and take to Miss Misscean. Any morning when pillows were stacked five high on Fullertoon's windowsill, a note would be waiting for him that night. The message was printed by Lieutenant Williams and placed in a small Beech Nut coffee can that had been part of her Red Cross comfort kit. Everyone involved in the transfer of information knew that discovery by the Japanese would mean torture and death, but they agreed to continue as long as the information was needed.[14]

Toward the end of September Lt. Ruby Bradley was brought to Santo Tomas from the prison camp in Baguio. She had decided months earlier that when the war came to an end, she wanted to be in a position to help the sick and wounded and therefore filed an application for transfer to Santo Tomas with little hope that her request would be granted. Finally, one evening at 1700 she was told she would leave for Santo Tomas the next morning. Lt. Beatrice

Chambers had not asked to go to Santo Tomas because she was reluctant to leave the area where she had been born and raised. As soon as she saw Bradley go out the gate of Camp Holmes, however, she regretted her decision to stay.[15]

One of the most frustrating things about being a prisoner of war in Santo Tomas was the realization that a POW or internee had little if any power over what happened to her. The Japanese often gave orders that seemed based on a whim and open to countermand by a mere change of mind. Faced with the lack of logic, consistency, and dependability in their daily lives, nurses spent considerable time alone and with each other trying to define some rationality in the winds of power that blew through their lives. An example of such an event occurred on 26 September 1943, when approximately 150 internees from Santo Tomas took part in a prisoner exchange between the United States and Japan. Lt. Eunice Young voiced the thoughts of most of the nurses when she wrote in her diary: "Still a mystery who picked the people to go. Well people leaving, while so many sick stay here."[16]

The nurses clung to hope as if it were a life preserver. Like tired swimmers, they held fast with both hands, praying that it and they would be carried into the future—one day at a time. Such determination kept them going in spite of the horrors and dangers that filled each day. It was that fortitude, that perseverance, that refusal to let go which on 9 November 1943 led Lt. Eunice Young to write in her diary: "Still wondering, 'When are the Americans coming?' A new moon so would be nice to have them come over any night now. The bedbugs and mosquitoes, the wormy mush and dewormed rice, the snooty civilians, the wooden beds, are all telling on my nerves. So hurry, Americans."[17]

The nurses would face many more discouraging situations before the camp was liberated. One such situation developed at 1500 on 14 November, when a strong typhoon hit the Philippines. Gale-force winds and heavy rain tore through Santo Tomas and Manila. Gas and electricity failed, the water supply was contaminated, and twenty-seven inches of rain fell in three days. Despite the terrible weather, sick and injured patients still needed care, and nurses still needed to get to work. The road between the main building where the nurses lived and Santa Catalina Hospital was about a block long and marked by a depression about twenty-five feet long and twenty-five feet wide. Four of the strongest men were assigned, two at each end of a thick manila hemp rope, to help the nurses across this depression. Lieutenant Ullom recalled that the water in the depression came up to their hips.

The nurses were wearing their shortest shorts and carrying their duty uniforms over their heads in accordance with an order by Captain Davison, despite the recent Japanese edict that women were not to wear shorts above their knees or slacks in camp. The action was a definite breach of Japanese orders and etiquette.[18] As Young stated, "Nothing happened because no Jap cared to tangle with the Major [Capt. Davison]."[19]

December saw the second anniversary of America's entrance into World War II. Many of the army nurses seemed surprised that they were still prisoners of war. "Two years today we went to war against Japan," Lieutenant Young wrote. "If anyone had told me that day that I would be here in this camp today, I wouldn't have believed it." Time, deprivation, and hunger were taking their toll on all POWs. Prices were going higher every day, and even if one had the money, many foods could not be bought. Eunice Young expressed the general frustration: "Impossible to buy sugar, and now no more given out on chow line. I know where there is some sugar, will have to see how good I am at thieving. (Hope after I get out of this mess I will never have to be without sugar.) Eggs are now 70 cents each, a tea cup of peanuts [$]1.10. Money doesn't go far and all this money will have to be paid back, that is if we ever get home to collect our pay. Our life these days is just one big 'if' after another."[20]

Despite the "ifs," nurses went on with their lives and work and kept their self-respect. All found it difficult to deal with their feelings concerning their captors, but some were more vocal than others. 2d Lt. Frances L. Nash was one of the vocal minority. One day while she was on duty in a clinic, a Japanese guard walked in and asked for medication for a bald spot on his head. Nash recalled: "I told him I was sorry, the Japanese would not give us any medication. He asked me where could he get some. I told him, 'The U.S.' I looked around and the doctor looked like he was about to faint. So, the guard bowed, I bowed, he thanked me and left. I asked the doctor, 'What's wrong?' He said, 'You know there is nothing to grow hair on his bald spots.' . . . I replied, 'You know he will never go to the States.' He replied, 'You will get us killed, one of these days, lying to them.' I said, 'Well, he left happy.' The doctor and I became good friends, but he said, 'I'll never understand you,' and shook his head. I don't think he ever forgot the bald spots."[21]

In mid-December, a group of internees found more than one hundred comfort kits that had been stored by the Japanese in the camp library and carried them outside and lined them up in long rows beside the main building. In response, Japanese military inspectors came to the camp and, while internees stood watching, they tore open the large cartons holding four food kits each and slashed into the individual kits. Stunned internees watched in horror as their captors thrust their knives into cans of salmon and meat and tore off all the labels to see if any messages were written on the reverse side.

Word of what the Japanese were doing to the food kits raced through the camp, and internees gathered quickly at the roped-off area where the "horror" was taking place. The Japanese opened each food kit and removed all cigarettes. Paper-wrapped prunes and raisins were left lying in the hot sun, where ants swarmed through them until late afternoon, when the plundered kits were finally given out.[22]

The meaning of those comfort kits to the POWs was exquisitely expressed by Lieutenant Young in her diary entry on 16 December 1943: "Today we received our kits at the hospital. American people at home will never know what a thrill it was to see American things after two years of this. Words cannot express our feelings. The Japs have promised us the cigarettes at a later date. The kits were all opened before we got them so we couldn't see how they had been packed, but even so, they are grand. Had a toasted cheese sandwich tonight, and grand cup of States coffee. We hear some people have already sold their kits for as much as 6000 pesos [$3,000]."[24]

This particular food kit would mean the difference between life and death for the army nurses and many internees. Unlike prisoners of war held by the Germans, who received comfort kits on a fairly regular basis, prisoners of the Japanese received only two or three comfort kits during their entire three and a half years of internment. Gorging, which took place in many German POW camps in the last year of the war, did not occur in Japanese camps because the food was not available. In addition, military nurses knew that stuffing a chronically empty stomach would lead to bloating and even death. This knowledge, combined with foresight and discipline, led them to dole out the contents over the next thirteen months and eighteen days.

Christmas 1943 was not so joyous as Christmas 1942, but at least there was still food and some presents for the children under age ten that had been handmade by internees. To everyone's disappointment, no one was allowed to visit in camp on Christmas Day. More than two thousand people arrived outside the main gate, hoping to be allowed to visit imprisoned relatives and friends, and were turned away by the imperious Japanese. It was the second Christmas for military nurses as prisoners of war. Young spoke for all the nurses when she wrote in her diary, "Surely it will be the last in here."[24]

The Entertainment Committee was very active from Christmas to the end of the year. On Christmas, the combined chorus of the camp led a "community sing" and performed Handel's *Messiah*. On New Year's Eve the Entertainment Committee put on *Cinderella* in the Little Theater Under the Stars. The cast consisted of 150 people, mainly young girls. The play ended at 2200, and most internees went to their quarters and were asleep long before midnight. Unlike New Year's Eve 1942, the streets around Santo

Tomas were quiet and there were no searchlights cutting through the night sky. A few private parties were held in the main building, but they too, were quiet. The eerie stillness hid the approach of further horrors and starvation that would seize the camp in the coming year.

9

Hunger in the Heart of Hell

Of all emotions mental and, of all feelings physical, hunger is unquestionably the most overpowering! I assure you, when you are hungry, you will do almost anything. Anything.

Major Josephine Nesbit Davis, USA, NC (Ret.)

The new year would bring drastic changes in the lives of those interned in Santo Tomas. On 10 January 1944, the commandant informed the Executive Committee that as of 6 January, Santo Tomas was under the direct authority of the War Prisoner Department commanded by General Morimoto. The Japanese military was now in charge of the internment camps in and around Manila. Radical changes took place in Santo Tomas after 1 February. Filipino doctors were no longer permitted to work in camp, and all internees housed in Sulfur Springs, Holy Ghost, and other hospitals or "special camps for the elderly" were brought into Santo Tomas. This change meant extra work for the army nurses who were now responsible for their care. The situation was made even worse by the Japanese military's order that only "extreme emergencies" could be sent to outside hospitals. The internees' morale went down considerably when the package line was closed permanently but bounced back somewhat when families were permitted to use the shanties again and the Japanese promised to supply fish and rice to the camp each month.[1]

Because of the expulsion of Filipino doctors from camp and the expected influx of internees from the now closed annexes, the Medical Board recommended that American doctors from nearby prisoner of war camps be transferred to Santo Tomas. It specifically requested one eye, ear, nose, and throat specialist; one tuberculosis specialist; three general practitioners; and two dentists.

In February conditions in the camp deteriorated considerably. In an attempt to improve the situation, the Executive Committee went against medical advice and allowed ducks to be kept in the shanty area with the hope that the ducks would provide food in the future.

With the military in charge of Santo Tomas, the camp was for all practical purposes cut off from the outside world. Lt. Earlyn Black, a twenty-five-year-old native of Groesbeck, Texas, recalled the effect the isolation had on the camp food supply and communications with the outside. Before this time many of the civilian internees received food from loyal Filipino servants who were permitted to bring it to the camp gate. These packages were frequently used to smuggle in news and personal notes, and now that avenue of contact was shut down.[2]

Fortunately, internees were still able to buy a few items at the vendors' market, and no one was yet experiencing real hunger. Nonetheless, money was scarce for the nurses and prices were still rising. A loaf of bread was selling for $1.80, and there was no guarantee how long it would be available. Cigarettes could no longer be purchased in the market or canteen, and smokers who had made purchases months earlier and stored them considered themselves lucky. Coffee drinkers were not as fortunate because it had disappeared from the chow line and was selling for forty pesos a cup at the Japanese-run canteen. Fresh milk and butter were something nurses could only dream about. Even old magazines reminded the captives of food. As Lieutenant Young said, "Ice cream, pie, steaks, apples, grapes and many other foods that we look at in 1941 magazine advertisements must be something foreigners in far away countries eat."[3]

In mid-February missionary doctors T.D. Stevenson, W.W.

McAnlis, and J.A. McAnlis were informed by the Japanese that they must either live and work outside or willingly be confined to Santo Tomas so they could treat the internees. They chose to live and work inside the camp.

On 18 February the Japanese commandant abolished the Executive Committee, replaced it with the Internee Committee, and appointed Carroll Grinnell as chairman. Earl Carroll and S.L. Lloyd were elected to the committee. The Japanese began delivering fish to Santo Tomas, small fish in poor condition. They were accompanied with a warning from the commandant that, "the fish, though small, had to be eaten" and that the prisoners of war in Bilibid had been "severely punished" when on one occasion they had buried, instead of cooked their fish. At first, fish arrived three times a week, and on one occasion, the fish cleaners found six toadfish, a poisonous variety of puffer fish, in three buckets of the daily ration. The commandant also informed the camp that the vegetable ration would cease at the end of February. After that, the produce grown in the camp garden, which was in the process of being established, would be substituted for vegetables in the ration. In an attempt to counteract these changes, the camp supplied internees with a small Philippine banana at breakfast and dinner. The fruit was a welcome change from fish and rice. Hunger was steadily becoming evident and malnutrition and starvation were only a matter of time.

For smokers, as the majority of the military and internees were in the early 1940s, cigarettes were almost as important as food. On 24 February Lieutenant Young wrote in her diary: "Blackie and I have 3 pkgs. of American cigs. left so we are smoking one a day to make them last as long as possible. We have rationed our Dobies [homemade] to 5 a day, which will make them last until May. By then surely something good will happen."[4]

As February wore on, the nurses were still hoping "something good would happen" when the Japanese stepped up unannounced inspections, thus adding to the danger of everyday life. Young felt this additional annoyance acutely when she wrote: "Big search going on in camp. Don't know what they want but must put this [diary] away. Hard to write from here as there are Japs all over the camp, never know when they are coming in."[5] Young knew only too well that getting caught with a diary would mean swift punishment, even death, at the hands of the Japanese military. Lt. Frances Nash, who also had kept a diary from the first days of her internment in Santo Tomas, destroyed it around this time, partly because of the constant need to rebury it after each entry, partly because her eyesight was deteriorating owing to the lack of adequate vitamins in the camp's diet.

The morale of the nurses received a boost on 26 February when three American doctors arrived from Cabanatuan, a prisoner of war camp about sixty miles north of Manila. The nurses were delighted to see old friends, Capts. Garnet Francis, Bloom, and Noell. Noell's wife was a civilian internee, and Francis was married to army nurse Earleen Francis. The morale of all medical personnel was dented a little when two days later the Japanese ordered the rodent control shed "closed and sealed." Because rodents could spread diseases through the camp, the order made no sense to anyone who had the internees' interests at heart.

It was also clear to all the nurses that the new roll call system ordered by the Japanese military to begin on 1 March was not intended to do the internees any good. Instead of room monitors taking roll and conveying the information to the Japanese, internees would now have to stand roll call twice a day, at 0800 and 1730, and be counted by Japanese soldiers. Lt. Hattie Brantley described the frustration caused by the new method: "We'd have to stand for hours while the Japs counted and recounted us. They never came up with the same numbers, and they couldn't count, so we'd have to stand there while they tried to reconcile their counts."[6]

The number of walls and fences around Santo Tomas was also subject to change. At one point, the Japanese ordered internees to begin construction on a bamboo fence around the camp, two meters from the inside of the wall. Not only did this order mean unnecessary work for internees who were growing weaker from malnutrition every day, but it would add to the feeling of isolation from the outside world.

Mounting frustration brought increased stress, and for smokers that meant a stronger craving for cigarettes. During the first week in March Lieutenant Young sold one can of milk for $75 and bought sixteen packages of Chesterfields for $76 dollars. Next to cartons of cigarettes for smokers, the packages given out by the Japanese on 3 March created the most excitement since the Christmas 1943 comfort kits. Young expressed the joy and suspicion those parcels brought to the internees: "What fun! Personal packages from home given out. Mine had a bathing suit. Guess my mother thinks I'm vacationing over here," she wrote. "These packages came in last November on the repatriation boat. Only about half the people in camp got one, although we know there must have been one for everybody. I consider myself just plain lucky to get mine."[7]

None of the nurses, including Eunice Young, knew, or could know, how hard their country had tried to get relief packages and supplies to them and their fellow prisoners of war in the Philippines. In June 1943 the *Prisoners of War Bulletin* first appeared. The bulletin was published by "The American National Red Cross for the Relatives of American Prisoners of War and Civilian Internees." In the last paragraph of the mission statement on page 1 of volume 1, number 1, the chairman of the American Red Cross said: "Channels of relief for American prisoners of war in Europe are operating smoothly. Despite difficulties which at times have appeared overwhelming, American Red Cross and the governmental agencies have continued negotiations seeking to open relief channels to our prisoners in the Far East. I assure you we will never abandon the effort to reach every prisoner of ours no matter where he may be held." One such effort had taken place in July 1942. A Swedish ship, the *Kanangoora*, with a neutral crew, was chartered and loaded in an American West Coast port with large quantities of food, clothes, medicines, and medical supplies. The ship stayed in port, fully loaded and ready to sail, until September, when the Japanese finally refused the Red Cross request for safe conduct. The Japanese government asserted that it could not guarantee safe conduct through waters in which active naval operations might take place. It was not until one year later, on 2 September, that the

M.V. *Gripsholm* sailed from Jersey City, New Jersey, for Marmagao, in Portuguese India, where the Japanese had agreed to an exchange of American and Japanese nationals set for 15 October 1943. The ship carried relief supplies furnished by the army, navy, and other United States agencies, valued at over $1.3 million. Over half of those supplies were earmarked for the Philippines.[8]

If Japan had allowed comfort kits and relief supplies into the Philippines on a regular basis, much of the hunger and starvation might have been avoided. Instead, by mid-March 1944, fights were breaking out among internees standing in long lines for hours to buy the few items of food available at exorbitant prices.

Food was now one of the main topics of conversation in camp, and internees wondered how long the Japanese would continue supplying their meager rations and just how bad the quality of that food would get in the coming months. Internees' attitudes toward food had to change drastically because they were obliged to eat what would have been considered garbage back home. Lt. Frances Nash expressed those changing attitudes: "I didn't want to starve, but did want to eat food that smelled good. One day we were eating cornmeal mush. Glad to get it. I saw a tiny mouse cooked in my mess kit. I pushed it aside. One of the nurses said, 'Nash, I'll give you some of mine.' I said, 'No, he was cooked in your mush, same as mine.'"[9]

Even the four thousand "fill-in-the-postcards" that were brought into Santo Tomas around 15 March did not take minds off food for long. The cards were preprinted with "I'm doing fine" messages, and internees were permitted to check the boxes and write a message not to exceed twenty-five words. All cards were censored so those written words had to be in keeping with the preprinted portion of the card. In their more than three years as prisoners of war in the Philippines, nurses were permitted to send such postcards only twice. Letters were sent to the POWs on a regular basis by families and friends, but only one or two letters were delivered to any nurse during her imprisonment. Thousands of letters must have been destroyed by their captors.

Early April brought several Japanese visitors to Santo Tomas, and the camp commandant "requested" that internees bow properly to all Japanese soldiers, but especially to officers. This repeated insistence on bowing greatly irritated the nurses, and they organized themselves to "strike back" as much as possible. Lt. Madeline Ullom expressed her feelings about those events: "By bowing, we were supposed to be showing our appreciation to the Imperial Japanese Army for their protection and kindnesses to us. You can imagine how well that went over with us. . . . Sometimes we'd space ourselves just so when we had to pass and bow to a guard. He no sooner straightened up from returning one bow, than another nurse would walk by and bow and he'd have to return her bow. Finally he'd just turn his back and ignore us as we passed. We all hated having to bow to the Sons of the Emperor."[10]

One of the April visitors to Santo Tomas unintentionally gave many of the internees a good laugh and a humorous memory that would bring a smile even years later. Ullom described that incident as only someone who experienced it could: "The Japanese Ambassador to Argentina happened to be going through Manila, and so he came into camp. We all went out to see what was going on. He was talking, and someone said, 'Can we ask some questions?' 'How is the war going?' 'Oh,' he says, 'We have advanced as far east from San Francisco as Chicago. There are some Indians there and the Indians are quite the fighters. They're having quite a little battle there with the Indians.' So we thought that was kind of funny. We all had poker faces. We didn't dare smile or laugh or say anything. He was talking to the whole camp. Everybody in camp who could walk, was down there to see who this fella was, and what he was doing."[11]

There was no humor in the words of the new commandant, Colonel Yoshie, who arrived on 26 April and ordered that all internees must sign a revised oath by 30 April or lose their classification as civilian internees. The forms provided to the internees were printed on both sides, one in English and one in Japanese. The original oath had required a pledge from each internee that he or she would follow the orders of the Japanese military authorities and under no circumstances would try to escape. The former Executive Committee had objected to the oath on the grounds that compliance with all Japanese orders might involve acts which the internees as loyal citizens of their own countries were not willing to commit. The revised oath deleted the pledge to comply with all orders of the Japanese military authorities, and most internees signed and noted their protest next to their signatures.[12]

Signing the revised oath did not add one aspirin or roll of gauze to the almost nonexistent medical supplies in POW and internment camps in the Philippines. Nurses and doctors were practicing their professions as best they could under the conditions. Fractures presented special problems because there was no plaster of paris in camp, and with hundreds of children to care for, broken arms were not unusual. Nurses used worn-out dresses and other discarded clothing to make the triangular bandages that bound broken bones.[13]

According to navy nurse Laura Cobb, Los Baños had its own special problems, not the least of which was how poorly equipped the hospital was with operating room linen that required hours of resterilization between surgeries. The clinic also was overwhelmed, handling from 170 to 200 cases a day.[14]

Dysentery plagued the internees and caregivers at both Los Baños and Santo Tomas. Patients with bacillary dysentery were treated with native-contrived serum and tea brewed from guava leaves; those with amebic dysentery, with carbarsene and emetine. Months of standing in line waiting to use the limited bathroom facilities and a chronically inadequate diet and foods such as cassava root, which contained elements that irritated the kidneys, caused urinary problems. The lack of urinary antiseptics led to chronic kidney conditions. At Los Baños Japanese callousness compounded those conditions. When Dr. Dana Nance requested permission to obtain his cystoscope and other genito-urinary instruments from Baguio, the Japanese military refused.[15]

Internees at Los Baños took extraordinary steps to combat one of their dietary deficiencies. Edwina Todd wrote later that "patients were so starved for fat they would beg for a dose of castor oil, drink an ounce and smack their lips. . . . Even rancid coconut oil seemed palatable."[16]

By the third week in May food was so scarce in Santo Tomas that if a nurse could buy one $2 egg a week, she considered herself fortunate. Sugar could no longer be bought at any price, and meat was a thing of the past. On 21 May 1944, Lieutenant Young marked her third birthday as a prisoner of war, and Carroll Grinnell and the Internee Committee discussed turning more unused land into gardens. Lack of food was now seriously affecting the internees' health. When the committee confronted Colonel Yoshie with this fact, the commandant denied there was any such problem. On 24 May Young wrote in her diary: "Commandant disagrees with Camp doctors about widespread loss of health and weight among internees; claims such losses are due to prolonged internment, separation of families, lack of regular communication. Refers to internees' letters to homeland, all of which show writers to be in good health! Advises eggs, sugar, milk, bananas, unavailable."[17]

Beginning in the last week of May unannounced roll calls and increasing numbers of searches added to the everyday misery of camp life. The rules for internees during these searches turned the process into a grotesque version of the children's game of statues. Lieutenant Ullom described the terrible toll these searches took on the nurses: "We would have to stand with one foot on one step, and one on the other, if that's where we were when the search started. We'd be that way for hours—until the Japanese said the search was over. It was really hard because often we had to really push ourselves just to climb a flight of stairs. We were weak from malnutrition and getting weaker every day. We made ourselves keep working, because we were American Army officers, and because people needed us."[18]

Despite the weakness and exhaustion, a solemn ceremony was held on 31 May at which internees read the names of the 249 fellow prisoners who had died since Santo Tomas opened.

May also brought drastic changes in the lives of prisoners of war and internees at Camp Holmes near Baguio. In November 1943, several months after Ruby Bradley's departure for Santo Tomas, a new Japanese commandant took charge. He treated the internees leniently, allowed greater quantities of food to come into the camp, and even issued passes so internees could go on walks near the camp. But when two internees escaped from camp and joined the guerrillas in May 1944, the attitude toward the remaining captives changed immediately. The lenient commandant was replaced by Commandant Oura, who carried out his duties with typical Japanese brutality. A twelve-foot-high, double barbed-wire fence was constructed around the camp. The outside fence was interlaced with bamboo sticks. As further punishment, food packages from outside were no longer permitted in camp and all money was confiscated and placed in the Bank of Taiwan.

Lt. Beatrice Chambers, the only military nurse in the camp, described several incidents that were the result of Japanese brutality and left indelible pictures in her mind. "They [the Japanese] took the men that were living or sleeping next to these men that escaped. They took them down to the locker [a food locker] and hung them by their thumbs," she said. "I tell you, they were wrecks when they came back."[19] Despite their torture, the Japanese did not find the escapees. They did, however, discover that the woman who slept on the wooden plank next to Chambers was the wife of a guerrilla. They removed her from the barracks and she was never seen again. The incident frightened Chambers so badly that she moved to another bed.[20]

Chambers described the brutality at Camp John Holmes against the woman who had been in charge of the Camp Fire Girls when Chambers was a child and a member of that troop: "The worst thing that happened up there [Camp Holmes] was, a missionary woman, a very fine woman, Mrs. Stein. She found out that the Filipinos were having a hard time with the Japs so she moved up north with her children [to help them]. Her husband stayed down below. She got in with a guerrilla force and was captured by the Japanese. They took her out because they figured she was a white woman, and she was the head of the guerrillas there. They took her and beheaded her in front of her children, and nobody knows what happened to those children unless they killed them. All gone. Everybody gone."[21]

Beatrice Chambers herself escaped death by a matter of inches while a prisoner in Camp Holmes. The fear that this incident engendered in Chambers and her fellow internees must have been severe. Knowing your captors could and would kill you on a whim is bad enough, but actually to be the target of a Japanese soldier who intends to kill you produces its own special brand of horror. Chambers recounted the incident:

> When we were first caught and sent to Camp John Holmes, I had a dog by the name of Ching. He was half Chow and half something else, but he was a fine dog. When the war hit, the GIs got him as a guard dog. He had like a khaki shirt on and a brown coat, and he was a watchdog. Well, when Baguio was made an open city, they let the dog go. He came right back to the nurses quarters. So he was sitting on the porch there, half starved like the rest of us, waiting for me. I yelled at him, he didn't see me, but he heard me. Once we were in the prison camp, we were behind chicken wire and other kind of wire and there was a hole in one of these wires there. I didn't see it, but the dog saw it. He came, and I tell you, I hears this whining, and there was Ching. What a wonderful reunion that was. We didn't realize what was going to happen. A Jap GI [soldier] came by with a bayonet fixed, and he saw me. He thought I was a boy that was going to get out of that hole with the dog. He came in and he made a lunge for me. Ching jumped up and caught the bayonet in his chest, and I got away. He killed Ching. That dog saved my life. That bayonet was for me. . . . There was a bunch of yelling and screaming going on. I managed to run off and get amongst all the prisoners. He lost sight of me. I mean it took him a little time to get the bayonet out of the dog. He threw the dog aside. That was the end of that. I've got a monument on one of the ranches for Ching. "Ching Chambers, heroic GI dog."[22]

A sense of humor helped Chambers survive. One incident involved a priest she had known as a child, who was now interned at Camp Holmes. "We had a Jesuit, a little Belgium padre, his name was Father Andreas," she said:

> His mind was up with the angels. He wasn't down in the gutter with the rest of us, to see all this hell going on. . . . The Japanese would come around and we'd all have to stand up and say, "Ohio" [Japanese for "good morning"]—Well, we had a big sergeant in the camp. He got fed up saying "Ohio," so he says to Father Andreas, "Father Andreas," he didn't say goddamn Jap because he couldn't say that to the padre. He said, "Father Andreas, when those Japs come around and we have to get up and say, "Ohio," instead of that you say "chicken shit."
> Father Andreas didn't know what chicken shit meant. He only knew French and the dialects. So, here come the Japs. Father Andreas gets up with his hands like a prayer, he gets up and bows to them, and says, "Chicken shit, chicken sheet." They didn't know what chicken shit [meant]. . . .
> I said, "Don't do that Father Andreas, they'll kill you for it." He asked, "Why, Beatrice?" "Because," I said, "that's a very bad term. You don't say that."
> Father Andreas got out in three months time, and the rest of us stayed over three years.[23]

There was little humor in Santo Tomas after June 1944. Conditions inside the camp became increasingly difficult. People were experiencing real hunger, and their perception of food was changing as a result. "We were so hungry that when we ate a banana, we ate the skin too," Lieutenant Brantley said. "Anything to fill up our empty stomachs."[24]

During the first week of June, one of the most terrifying experiences of the army nurses' captivity took place. The Japanese ordered that everyone in Santo Tomas be inoculated against "plague." Since there had been no cases of plague in camp, the order aroused fear and suspicion among doctors and nurses about the intentions of their Japanese captors. Lt. Madeline Ullom recalled that experience:

> Apparently they were studying [experimenting with] the plague, and they wanted to get rid of us, liquidate us. [This rumor had gained more weight as it became obvious that the war was not going well for the Japanese.] They came along and they said, "Everybody has to take this [medication or inoculation]. There is an epidemic of plague," they said. They gave us these vials of plague medication and we were to give everyone in camp a shot. I was often working in the clinic as well as in the hospital and I was to give a half a cc [cubic centimeter], I think. Everything was written in Japanese. I was petrified because I didn't know if that was plague or something else—or what it was. Everybody in camp had to get a shot. And I tell you, I was petrified, having to give all these shots to people. And so in the next couple days when they were still walking around and all right, I breathed a little easier. I got it myself. All these guards were around you with their guns and their bayonets [to make sure the medication was given].

Ullom asked questions about that "plague" medication when she returned to the United States. "From what I could find out later, they had decided they weren't going to try to kill everybody with the plague," she said. "So, maybe some of these bugs that they had developed had gotten out in or near camp, and they didn't want it to be discovered that they were planning to kill us. They probably changed their minds before some of what they developed got out, so they had everyone inoculated."[25]

Considering that the Japanese did not go out of their way to get desperately needed medications and medical supplies for the internees at Santo Tomas and that they confiscated most of what the Red Cross sent for use by the camp, it seems out of character for them to spend money on or use Japanese-made medication for "the good" of the camp population. Ullom's conjecture is supported by documents discovered in the early 1990s and analyzed by Ika Toskija and Yoshimi Yoshiaki at the Research Library of the Japanese Defense Agency in Tokyo confirming that the Japanese planned to use biological weapons in the southwest Pacific during World War II. Japan first planned to use biological agents in the Philippines by releasing one thousand kilograms of plague-infected fleas on U.S. and Filipino troops on Bataan. While the biological weapons were being prepared, General King surrendered Bataan and the plan was abandoned. Fleas were a favorite vector of the Japanese in delivering plague to an enemy, and rats were a preferred delivery system. The closing and sealing of the rodent shed in Santo Tomas in February 1944 takes on a more ominous tone when viewed in this light. The willingness of the Japanese to use biological agents was demonstrated in the Jinhua area of Zhejiang Province of China in June and July 1942 when they used plague and dysentery to retaliate against the Chinese for helping American plane crews under the command of Jimmy Doolittle, who landed in China after their attack on Tokyo and Naggoya. The Japanese were appalled when the wind carried some of the pathogens over Japanese troops and killed more than seventeen hundred of their own soldiers.[26]

In addition to this biological warfare, the Japanese used POWs to experiment with malaria immunizations. An American former POW, Capt. John Murphy, gave testimony concerning such experiments in July 1945, when he and 1st Class Airman Palmer were injected with an untried serum concocted by Dr. Einosuke Hirano of the Japanese army. Hirano and Dr. Fushida of the Sixth Field Kempeitai had experimented with malaria immunizations in 1943 after Japanese supply lines to Rabaul were cut and the supply of quinine, desperately needed by malaria-ridden Japanese troops, had been depleted. Although we cannot confirm that the injections given to the POW military nurses in Santo Tomas were biological agents or experimental serum, we can be sure that neither action was beyond the ethics and morals of the Japanese military.[27]

The one bright spot in June came into camp in the pages of the *Manila Tribune*. Lieutenant Young wrote in her diary: "Today's paper announced the invasion of France. Everyone in camp very excited! I had a drink of rice wine to celebrate the grand news. We sure have a lot of catching up to do when we get out of here. Maybe X-mas!" [28]

Three days later, Japanese military authorities ordered the internees to construct a barbed wire fence one meter high on top of the one-and-a-half-meter-tall bamboo fence that stood ten meters from the camp wall. When the Internee Committee refused to tell the internees to work on building these fences without a written order, the Japanese provided one to the committee and the fences were constructed.

Given the meager diet of the internees, ordering them to do physical labor was cruel. From May through the first half of September, the Japanese failed to deliver the rations they had promised. By 23 June, eggs, when they were available, were selling for $2.10 each. Deliveries of rice and corn dwindled to almost nothing, and the Japanese substituted camotes, a very poor variety of sweet potato that was grown in the Philippines. When the camotes were peeled and the bad ones removed, they were less than one-sixth of the weight of the rice that had been promised. In addition, the camotes were irritating to the normal digestive tract and caused many problems for those who had suffered from dysentery and other intestinal maladies. As a result, the Internee Committee reluctantly decided to draw on the camp's sparse reserves of rice for as long as they lasted.

The fish promised by the Japanese was a great disappointment. The few large fish in the best condition were given to the hospitals for patients. The chow lines usually received small fish that were more bone, head, and tail than meat. An even smaller fish known as "sap-sap" was delivered with greater frequency. Sap-sap were native fish ranging from two to three inches in length. These fish were tremendously difficult to clean, and more often than not, they were simply thrown into cooking pots and served as an unappetizing soup. The condition of the sap-sap was not helped by the lack of refrigeration and ice and the fact that the Japanese military were in no hurry to deliver it to the enemies of Japan. On at least one occasion, the entire supply had to be discarded as not fit for human consumption.

One of the most important items of food, given the extreme heat of the tropics, was salt. The only salt available was rock salt that was very different from the granulated variety the nurses had used years ago in the luxury of the Army and Navy Club and in their own dining facilities. Animal fats and cooking oils were also nearly nonexistent. The ration, originally twenty grams, was soon reduced to ten and then to five grams. Jars of cold cream that had been tucked away made their appearance as cooking staples. Nurses began to speculate on the use of camp food reserves to augment their already starvation rations. Most agreed that they were glad they did not have to make the decision.

July opened to memories of Fourth of July picnics before the war. The only Fourth of July entertainment the Japanese would allow was a costume party for the children. When the musical broadcast of the evening ended, the children marched from their playhouse to the plaza in columns of two. They were dressed as sailors, soldiers, cowboys, and Indians. The assembled internees suddenly realized that a small girl at the head of the column was carrying a twelve-inch hand-painted American flag. It was the first time the American flag had been displayed in the camp, and people rose to their feet as it passed. Despite this act of patriotism, the internees' morale received several bad blows during July.

On 5 July, in an apparent effort further to isolate the camp, the Japanese ordered that laundry could no longer be sent outside camp. Because of the lack of laundry equipment and soap and the approximately three hundred sets of hospital bed linens to wash, this new obstacle to basic cleanliness would place an additional heavy burden on this beleaguered population, since all would potentially be affected.

Another order announced during the last week in July surprised internees and delivered another blow to their morale. The city garbage truck would no longer be allowed to come into the camp, so they would have to bury any garbage that could not be fed to the pigs and ducks. The new edict placed additional, unnecessary physical demands on the malnourished internees and ended the small amounts of food, messages, and money that previously had been smuggled into camp, hidden on the truck.

On the first day of August, a particularly stunning blow fell. The internees learned that all money in camp—private, trust, and camp funds—must be surrendered immediately for deposit in the Bank of Taiwan. Individuals were permitted to retain only fifty pesos.[29]

They would thus have less money to buy extras that were more and more important in view of the starvation diet furnished by the Japanese. On the fifth day of August, the Internee Committee presented three written communications to the commandant. One letter stated the opinion of the Health Committee that the Japanese food policy would result in starvation for the camp's population. The second letter protested the takeover by the Japanese military of a garden plot cleared by the internees. The seizure was seen as another step by the Japanese in bringing about the deaths of the internees through starvation. The third letter requested that the allowable individual sum of money per month be raised from fifty to one hundred pesos.

Food deliveries by the Japanese became spasmodic and were usually 10 percent underweight. After July, the fish that arrived in camp were dilis, two inches or less in length, salted and dried in the sun as soon as they were caught. Dilis were not cleaned and had an overpowering, unpleasant odor. Few internees would eat them at first, but as hunger grew worse, they ignored the bad odor and consumed them gratefully as a soup or warmed whole.

At this point the Internee Committee decided to use the camp reserves of canned meat and canned vegetables. They estimated that the reserves would be exhausted by the end of October and hoped that they would be liberated by then. The camp was shocked when on 16 August, the commandant, Lieutenant Colonel Hayashi, canceled an order for vegetables placed by the Internee Committee. Hayashi and his right-hand man, Lieutenant Abiko, told the committee, "The internees were greedy and selfish and desirous of buying heavily in the open market outside, thereby depriving starving Filipinos of much needed food." In truth, relatively few vegetables were needed for four thousand internees compared to the needs of a large city. [30] The entire ration of fish delivered on 19 August by the Japanese army was unfit for human consumption and was fed to the ducks. The camp diet had degraded to the point that signs of malnutrition and starvation were becoming more evident. The camp's corned beef reserve was doled out at a rate of one twelve-ounce can for four people twice a week. This gave internees six ounces of corned beef a week and did much for morale even though it probably did not have a great effect on their physical health.

On 27 August, the Japanese announced that all "enemy aliens" would be brought into the camp from the Hospicio de San José, the Remedios Hospital, and the Philippine General Hospital. Approximately two hundred people from these institutions arrived on the last day of the month. Thirty were women, and many of the remaining 170 were old men in very poor health. Many of these new internees could not stand in chow lines and required nursing care.

An average of only 27.4 grams, less than one ounce per person per day, of meat and fish were provided to the camp by the Japanese army for the month of August.

Beginning in late August, thefts in camp increased greatly. The largest numbers and most frequent thefts were from the kitchens, the food lines, and the vegetable preparation areas. Since the crimes were petty, about the most that could be done was to dismiss the thief from food preparation or food service.

This type of crime was committed by men who carried away cooked rice by stuffing it into their pockets and by women who were peeling and cleaning vegetables, but carried off the peelings to cook for themselves or their families. It was common to see men and women going through vegetable refuse in hopes of finding something they could add to a soup or use as an extra piece of food. In his book *The Story of Santo Tomas*, A.V.H. Hartendorp states: "It was becoming very apparent to what degree plain honesty, ordinary decency, self-respect, community feeling, and all the higher moral values are dependent on the maintenance of the narrow margin between having enough to eat and not having enough to eat. Man is first an animal, and an animal is mostly stomach."[31]

Years later Josephine Nesbit Davis spoke to this point in a letter to Dorothy Starbuck, the director of veterans benefits for the Veterans Administration:

> Our situation gave us problems never faced by any group of Nurses—face to face with a determined adversary and dedicated enemy who loved especially to "lord it over Americans". . . . Add to it that intangible of trying to contain ourselves while the other, more affluent civilians prepared additional food. It took every bit of willpower to learn to accept what was inevitable: They were not going to share with us—and that was that. It was a very difficult situation to accept. . . .
>
> Our Junior Nurses were (pardon my frankness) literally "sitting on a gold mine" insofar as personal needs and wants were concerned. It would have been easy to succumb to the temptations which we encountered; extra food, particularly, to make life a little easier, was within easy reach. Heavens above and alone knows what might have been the consequences. . . . Hunger knows no bounds. . . . What held us together, physically and emotionally, was PRIDE. We were proud of the fact we were U.S. Army Nurses.[32]

In September the food situation got even worse. On 13 September, the commandant announced that because of problems in transporting rice, the camp's rice ration was cut from 400 to 300 grams per day. The rice ration was cut again on 19 September, from

300 to 250 grams a day (9.7 ounces). In response, the Internee Committee authorized the use of 40 grams of rice per person per day from the camp reserves.

Despite malnutrition and starvation, the internees' morale soared on 21 September. Lieutenant Young recorded that day in her diary: "Day of all days! Our first bombing at 9:30 this A.M. We could see the American planes, 7 were counted. The anti-aircraft fire was bad for us here. The camp wild with excitement. . . . 3 P.M. They are back again—full force—the shrapnel is falling near us. I hope our boys know this is Santo Tomas. They bombed the harbor and the airfields. Large fires can be seen burning. The Filipinos have my sympathy."[33]

During the first week in October, word got around the camp that the two hundred ducks belonging to the internees were to be killed and served for a supper before mid-October. The ducks had been fed mainly on camp garbage, and many of them were as malnourished as the internees. Anyone who expected to see duck on his plate was disappointed. The duck was ground and mixed into fried rice, which tasted faintly of duck. On the blackboard that announced the menu for the day were the following words: "Two hundred ducks—293 lbs. gross, 190 lbs, net; the ducks were starving, too."[34]

In an attempt to ensure the equitable distribution of food in camp, the Internee Committee appointed a new group to the camp patrols and assigned it to patrol food supply and preparation areas. By the second week in October internees were receiving approximately six ounces of food a day: Two ounces of mush for breakfast, two ounces of rice for lunch, and two ounces of rice and gravy for supper. Many of the nurses wondered if people at home had any idea of what it was really like to be hungry.[35]

In yet another callous display of unconcern for the safety of prisoners of war and internees, four truckloads of Japanese soldiers arrived in camp on 9 October and set up a series of tents in the southwest garden area beside the road. Heavy equipment and block and tackle were set up in front of the education building. Internees were instructed to stay out of the areas where Japanese soldiers were working. The commandant further ordered that all firewood be moved out of the west pavilion because it was to be used as a Japanese dormitory.

Obviously the Japanese were trying to safeguard their troops from American bombing raids by billeting them inside an internment camp. A further travesty of justice and honor occurred when the Japanese used several towers inside the camp for signal towers, thereby endangering the entire camp population. Would a "friendly" bomb fall on the camp because of the Japanese actions? This question only added to the stress caused by the insecurity about food. How many people would starve to death before the Americans finally came? Would the Japanese exterminate the camp's population before the Americans could liberate them?

In the face of starvation and unimaginable stress among the internees, Lieutenant Abiko supervised the initial formal bowing classes during the first week of November. Three hundred monitors were brought to the hospital compound and instructed in the proper method of bowing. The internees were told that they would be instructed by the monitors over the next three days in the art of "showing respect." Those who did not learn or who did not bow properly after the classes would be punished. Roll calls became an occasion when internees would bow in unison to the Japanese officers and have their "respect" returned with a salute. More often than not, Lieutenant Abiko was the one accepting their "show of respect," and he became irretrievably associated with the harping insistence that internees humble themselves in this way. Bowing to the Japanese was not only aggravating to the nurses, it was physically difficult for them. Everyone was skeleton-thin, and they could no longer climb a flight of stairs without stopping several times to rest.

In mid-November, the camp food reserves were all but exhausted. Frederic Stevens's description of the conditions brought about by starvation creates images that are unforgettable.

The shortage of food resulted in a number of features symptomatic of semi-starvation. Domestic animals were killed and eaten in some cases; of the flocks of pigeons

nesting about the Main Building, only a few strays remained by December; leaves and roots of unaccustomed
plants were cooked for food; while inability or disinclina-
tion to withstand, even at this stage, a comparatively
empty stomach led to the highly dangerous and disgusting practice of salvaging condemned vegetables and other
decaying matter from the camp garbage. After camotes
were peeled or vegetables cleaned at the dining shed
benches, numbers of women and children arrived to pick
up and carry away the refuse. Children hung about the
food processing shed in the hope of picking up a stray
camote or piece of squash. Orders had to be given putting an end to this practice.[36]

Despite their starvation, the nurses maintained a sense of humor. Lieutenant Brantley recalled an incident involving one of the
missionary doctors: "I don't remember that anybody had an animal
with them, but strays got into camp. An old cat got into the hospital
all the time, and we'd always tried to catch him. One night I heard
this terrible ruckus and I went downstairs to investigate. Doctor
Smith, an old missionary doctor was down there in the [hospital]
kitchen, and he was dressing him [the cat]. I said, 'Dr. Smith, what
are you doing, surgery?' And he said, 'Hell, no, I'm going to eat this
bastard!' He'd gotten pretty crude by this time. You get that way when
you don't have anything to fill your stomach."[37]

Another source of humor for the nurses was the commandant's
order on 15 November that fifty books at a time from the camp
library were to be submitted to the commandant's staff for his
"chop" or mark of official approval. The order seemed incongru-
ous in such a serious situation. Brantley managed to get a smile
out of it. "Here we were starving and they were worried about library books. They removed many history books for the dumbest
of reasons. Some they excluded because they stated that Balboa
had discovered the Pacific Ocean. The Japs said, 'He did not! It was
there all the time.'"[38]

An order by the commandant in mid-November was no laughing matter. He pointed out that there were "high growing" crops in the forbidden area, within twenty meters of the wall. The offending crops were papaya trees, and the commandant ordered that they be removed immediately or they would be destroyed. This order in the face of starvation within the camp only added to the pent-up anger the internees felt for their captors.

Similar conditions existed at Los Baños and are described by Lt. Edwina Todd:

By November 1944 weakness was a cause of worry to the hospital staff. Our rubberkneed corpsmen were no longer able to push the "Camp gearney" used as a stretcher for patients, carpenters were no longer able to make coffins, the grave-diggers to dig graves, the nurses literally pulled themselves up the stairs. . . . When you bent to rub a patient's back you wondered if you could straighten up again. You fell down a couple of times en route to and from work. Your hand shook as you gave an injection as well as when you assisted in the OR or gave medication. The surgeon was in a similar state. Through [though] loathe to admit it you were often incontinent. As soon as the desire to void occurred the act was a fact, especially at night. This was demoralizing as well as rendering one less efficient. We realized that it was no longer a question of our liberators coming but our survival until they arrived.[39]

The camp was approaching a new level of horror. People were suffering from beriberi, and nurses and doctors realized that many were beyond saving even if the Americans arrived that day to liberate them. Lieutenant Ullom remembered those people: "There were two kinds of beriberi, dry and wet. With the dry, you just shriveled up and kind of turned to dust as you wasted away. The wet was much more serious and deadly. Men got the wet type more because they needed more protein. You could see a man one evening and he'd look normal [given camp conditions]. You could see the same man the next day and he'd be all bloated. His face, hands and legs would be several times normal in size. You knew then that he didn't have long to live. His heart would enlarge too, and he'd get pulmonary edema, and die of congestive heart failure."[40]

The condition of the camp population was obvious to the trained eyes of doctors and nurses. The same compassion and empathy that had led them into the medical profession pulled at their hearts and intellects. "People in camp are really hungry," Lieutenant Young said. "I hate to see the expressions on their faces, especially families with children. The Japs will not listen to any appeal for more food. I can't imagine what's going to happen to this camp if help doesn't arrive soon."[41]

During the last weeks in November, the Japanese brought more equipment into Santo Tomas, and nurses and internees wondered what was in store for them. It was an unintended kindness that they were not told. Unintended kindness was the only humane treatment the Japanese showed their prisoners in the Philippines. Even holidays that were once looked to with anticipation began to blur in the minds of a population racked with devastating malnutrition. Eunice and Blackie had two cans of Spam left. One they shared for Thanksgiving, the other they saved for Christmas dinner.

By December 1944 internee deaths were increasing with each passing day. At Santo Tomas six to seven prisoners died each day from starvation and at Los Baños, one to two. All of the living were ravaged by the effects of malnutrition and starvation. Eighty percent had beriberi. An obsession with food led to a new camp activity, trading recipes. Patients with feet swollen from beriberi and scurvy would discuss foods and recipes. It was a favorite form of rationalization.[42]

Rationalization about starvation was impossible for Lieutenant Nash. She described the hunger she witnessed: "The look of hunger is unmistakable, but the pain of hunger is indescribable. I saw my friends' faces with the skin drawn tight across the bones, their eyes sunken, unnaturally bright, and deeply circled. Because of general malnutrition and vitamin deficiency, I was always bordering on beriberi, and I had amoebic dysentery twice. Hunger makes one constantly dizzy and causes a severe basal headache that never leaves. My ankles were swollen, I never knew what it was to feel well. By December 1943, I had been without vitamins so long that I could not read a line of print. The letters swam together."[43]

Children reacted to starvation by begging candy, sugar, and tobacco from the Japanese soldiers. To address this problem, the commandant followed the ancient proverb "Out of sight, out of mind" and ordered that all children were to be kept away from the Japanese kitchen and office. In addition, the children would suffer further deprivations at Christmas. It was clear to everyone that there would be no entertainment or presents for the children this year. On 20 December the Japanese cut the rice ration per individual from 210 to 200 grams a day.

On 23 December, the Kempeitai, the brutal Japanese equivalent of the feared and notorious Nazi Gestapo, arrived in camp with a platoon of soldiers and searched the hospital compound and the main building. Without any explanation, Carroll C. Grinnell, Clifford Larsen, A.F. Duggleby, and E.E. Johnson were arrested, questioned in the commandant's office, then placed in jail.

Christmas Eve brought several surprises to Santo Tomas. Leaflets bearing a Christmas message from the Allied forces were dropped on the camp. Prisoners hid as many of the leaflets as they could grab before the Japanese stepped in and said all leaflets must be turned in to the commandant's office. The message on the leaflets read: "The Commander-in-Chief, the officers and the men of the American Forces of Liberation in the Pacific wish their gallant allies, the people of the Philippines, all the blessings of Christmas and the realization of their fervent hopes for the New Year. Christmas 1944."[44] Every internee the Japanese found with the leaflet was sentenced to seven days in jail.

On Christmas Eve, by decision of the Internee Committee, each internee received one spoonful of jam and fifteen grams of sweet chocolate. Everyone over age sixteen received five cigars and four cigarettes. Eunice and Blackie cut up the cigars and made cigarettes with the tobacco. For paper, they used the packaging around cotton and ended up with blue hand-rolled cigarettes.

One might conclude that nurses and internees had little to be thankful for on Christmas 1944, but Lieutenant Young wrote cheerfully: "Had choc. and bread with jam for breakfast for Blackie and I. Fried rice to-nite and what a difference a full stomach makes in people's morale. We had Minnie [Breese] with us to-nite. We opened a can of Spam, a can of grape jelly and what a meal we had. Everyone excited over leaflets dropped in camp last night, the message was real nice, a real Xmas present from outside."[45]

Paper was not the only thing that the Allies were dropping over Manila. Bombings occurred sporadically over the next months, and blackout conditions, mandated by the Japanese, continued in effect.

As bad as things were for the nurses in Santo Tomas in December, conditions were worse at Camp Holmes. Lt. Beatrice Chambers and her fellow internees had been moved by truck to Bilibid Prison in Manila on 28 December 1944. They arrived at 0200. The Japanese had deliberately left all camp supplies, including food, behind at Camp Holmes, and the newly arrived prisoners immediately found that Bilibid was plagued by sanitation problems. The camp was filthy and overrun by insects, rats, and lice. There were no mops, brooms, or other tools for cleaning. Prisoners had to scrape filth from the floor with their own hands. When it seemed things could get no worse, their food ration was dropped to two hundred grams (eight ounces) a day, beginning 1 January 1945.

On New Year's Day 1945 a Japanese officer was reported to have said, "The white population at Santo Tomas was never a problem for the Japanese, as it was believed that an extremely restricted diet and disease would take care of the situation in due course."[46] Starvation was exacerbated when on 1 January 1945, the rice ration at Santo Tomas was cut to 110 grams (about four ounces) per person per day.

On 5 January, the Kempeitai took Grinnell, Duggleby, Johnson, and Larsen out of the camp. The next day the Japanese burned their own records and a Japanese officer broadcast his good-bye and best wishes over the loudspeaker system. The same evening at roll call, it was announced that the Japanese were still in charge of the camp.

Air raids continued day and night over Manila and surrounding areas. On 8 January, internees saw an American bomber receive a direct hit from anti-aircraft guns. The plane burst into flames, and internees watched as the crew bailed out and parachuted toward the ground.

Internees were angered and concerned when on 11 January the commandant's office complained again of the "laxity" of the camp in "showing respect." Showing respect for the Japanese was not high on the priority list of a starving population, but each person realized bowing was an absolute necessity. Lt. Madeline Ullom recalled her concerns: "I used to worry that if I bent over to bow, I'd just keep right on going. We were all so weak. Or maybe I wouldn't be able to straighten up again."[47]

By mid-January, a typical day's routine, not including surprise searches or extra roll calls, was as follows:

Morning	*Afternoon/Evening*
7—Reveille (music over loudspeaker)	1–3—Quiet period (He who sleeps, eats.)
8—Roll call to 9:30, breakfast (after roll call)	4:00—Dinner
9:30 to 11:30—No movement about camp except in groups specially designated	5:30 to 6:30—Roll call, then sit outside on plaza
	6:30—Curfew, everybody inside
11:30—Camp information period	7:00—Lights out[48]
11:45—Lunch, if any	

On 14 January, the Internee Committee asked the commandant's office where Grinnell, Duggleby, Johnson, and Larsen were being kept and why they were in the custody of the Kempeitai. The commandant told the committee he could not answer either question. On 18 January, the Internee Committee again inquired as to the whereabouts of the four arrested men and requested their return. They also asked to be told what charges, if any, were preferred against them. There was no response from the Japanese.

Starvation was ravaging the camp population. Those who could still perform their assigned duties wondered how long they would be able to function. Lieutenant Young reflected the trepidation of all the nurses: "Our chief concern is food. People are actually dying from starvation. We live from one meal to the next as we are hungry all the time. Everyday one or more brought into the hospital after having fainted from hunger. Haven't the energy to write much for days . . . but we have to keep going to take care of the others. Words can never describe how miserable we feel. Will appreciate the simple things of life, if we get out—just never to be hungry again!"[49]

On 28 January, the Japanese medical officer in charge of prison camps in the Philippines, Dr. Nogi, told two of the camp physicians, Dr. Smith and Dr. Stevenson, that eight recent death certificates listing malnutrition or starvation as a cause of death were an insult to the Japanese army. Dr. Nogi said in effect, "Things are tough all over," and he wanted Dr. Stevenson to change the cause of death on the certificates. Dr. Stevenson was given until 29 January, when he refused to change the certificates, resigned as chief medical officer, and was thrown into the camp jail.

In her 29 January 1945 diary entry, Lt. Eunice Young noted that so many internees were dying from malnutrition that someone was always gasping a last breath each time she walked through her ward. Adding to this stress were the sounds of almost continuous explosions of bombs falling around Manila for the past several days.[50]

Although internee deaths were increasing every day, the Japanese announced that the dead would no longer be taken outside camp for burial. Bodies would be collected and buried in mass graves inside Santo Tomas. The rats that had proliferated since the Japanese closed and sealed the rodent control shed in February were also starving and turned their hunger on the dead. One can well imagine the picture those horrors painted in the minds of the nurses. "The people were dying and we were having to keep their bodies in the hospital," Lieutenant Ullom said. "There were loads and loads of rats; some of them were a foot long, and some of them were bigger, and that's not counting their tails. Finally we had to have a cemetery right in Santo Tomas, because the rats were eating the fingers and toes off of the bodies. It was things like that went on every day—every day."[51]

At the end of January Lieutenant Abiko notified the Internee Committee that all medical certificates excusing internees from roll calls were canceled. Everyone, regardless of condition, must stand roll call. Abiko also pointed out that internees were again not showing proper respect for Japanese officers and soldiers and insisted that they do so beginning immediately or face punishment.

In the opening days of February, the Japanese took several brutal steps to feed themselves. On 1 February, the Japanese ordered several internees to kill the two remaining carabaos in camp. The meat was to be used by the Japanese, who refused to shoot the beasts. The internees tied the animals to a tree, blindfolded them, and tried to kill them with a hammer. When this did not work, the doomed beasts were killed with two blows from a large sledgehammer. Groups of children who had stood off, witnessing the slaughter, watched the animals being butchered and carried away. Then the children rushed to the spot to fill their cups with anything remaining that might be eaten.[52]

On 2 February, the Japanese stripped any remaining fruits and vegetables from the internees' gardens.

In his book *Santo Tomas Internment Camp*, Frederic Stevens presents us with a stark and harrowing picture:

The internees presented the appearance of an army of walking skeletons. Pipe-stem legs seemed scarcely able to bear the bodies above them; arms were thin and scrawny; the skin wrinkled, without elasticity, hung down in folds; the men wearing no shirts showed prominently a corrugation of ribs like washboards. They walked about with a listless air, staring at the ground, scarcely giving a glance at those who chanced to pass them. This Santo Tomas "stare" was characteristic. The girls still kept appearances with their lipstick and rouge, but there was no hiding the fact that they were all pretty thin. . . . The appearance of the camp inmates filled one with horror and pity. Help must come to save the camp, and help did come on February 3rd.[53]

10

Liberation

*Suddenly, and with stark delineation, the full impact of
what it means to be a prisoner of war entered into and
became our reality. The loss of freedom is, perhaps one of
the most difficult things any American, or any citizen of a
democracy, can endure. Freedom is after all, the essential
ingredient of democracy. . . . I and my fellow POWs, the
survivors of Bataan and Corregidor, are proud to be
counted in that long line of patriots, who have been willing
to risk everything—for the right to be free.*

Lt. Col. Madeline Ullom, USA, NC (Ret.)

During the day on 3 February 1945, there were sounds of explosions and intermittent gunfire in and around Manila. The sky was filled with smoke that rose from fires south and east of Santo Tomas. Inside the camp the Japanese were hurriedly packing or burning whatever records they had not previously destroyed. Nurses were going about their assigned duties and daily routine when Lt. Minnie Breese glanced up and saw the sky black with American planes. "I knew they weren't Japanese. They had a different sound. . . . We had a bet going on. Who was going to make it first. The First Cavalry, the Marines, or the vultures. And we thought for a while, the vultures were going to win."[1]

About 1700, ten American planes flew over Santo Tomas. One of the aircraft left the formation and dropped something into the camp. Madeline Ullom recalled that exciting incident and the fateful message: "The pilot flew real low over Santo Tomas and dropped his goggles. A piece of paper was around the lens and it said, 'Christmas is here. We'll be in today or tomorrow.'" The news spread like wildfire, and the camp was riveted with excitement.[2]

At 1800 the loudspeaker carried the announcement that all internees were to go to their rooms for the night. They were ordered to observe a total blackout and to stay away from the windows. They were also warned that anyone seen looking out of a window would be shot.

Internees sat in darkness in rooms and corridors discussing whether the Japanese had locked them in their buildings in preparation for disposing of them. But no matter what topic they started to discuss, they ended up talking about food. Even the thought of death was not strong enough to overpower the starvation that wracked their bodies and minds. The nurses' rooms looked out on the large iron gates in front of Santo Tomas, and the nurses stood back and stared out the windows. Madeline Ullom recalled that night: "We could smell gasoline, and hear a steady rumbling sound moving toward Santo Tomas. . . . At first we were worried that they might be Jap tanks coming to finish us off."[3]

Between 2030 and 2100, American tanks entered the camp. Madeline Ullom described the long-awaited deliverance: "We watched as the tanks crashed through the gates and rolled to a stop in front of the main building. An American soldier walked in front of the tanks. . . . The whole plaza was bright with the tanks' searchlights. The soldier called out, 'Hi folks! Are there any Americans in there?' Suddenly the camp was alive with voices calling out from everywhere. 'You'd better believe it!' 'We're in here!' 'We're Americans!' Suddenly everyone was running downstairs to get outside. The doors were locked, so I think we just broke through them. We were like a wave engulfing the tanks and American soldiers. Some people were shouting, 'They're here!' Others were yelling, 'We're free!' Someone started singing, 'God Bless America' and between laughing and crying, we all joined in."[4]

The soldiers shot flares into the air, and the plaza in front of the main building was as bright as in daylight. American troops poured into the camp, and nurses saw the first healthy Americans they had seen in more than three years. "They looked like giants compared to us, the Filipinos, and Japanese," Lieutenant Brantley said. "We were all so puny and dried up, and these soldiers looked like oil was coming out of their skin. They looked so healthy."[5]

The soldiers had fought their way to Santo Tomas under direct orders from Gen. Douglas MacArthur. MacArthur had reason to believe that the Japanese were planning to kill their prisoners, and he directed the First Cavalry and the Forty-fourth Tank Division to fight their way to Santo Tomas without securing the areas they went through. He further ordered them to take their wounded with them instead of setting up aid stations. Truckloads of wounded were brought into camp.

POW nurses and doctors set up a hospital in the main lobby and immediately went to work. There was only one doctor and several medics with the troops, so the participation of internment camp medical personnel was essential if the wounded were to live. The soldiers were treated and placed in three rooms off the make-shift emergency hospital. The rooms had previously been the home for women internees, and the men were placed in the beds amid clothes hanging on T-shaped poles over one end of each bed. While their wounded were being taken care of by the POW army nurses and physicians, including Dr. Stevenson, who just had been liberated from the camp jail, the American soldiers asked the internees where the Japanese were hiding. Internees pointed toward the education building at the same moment internees inside the building called out from the second floor windows, "The Japs won't let us out! They're holding us hostage!"

At this time Commandant Hayashi sent two members of the Internee Committee out of the education building to negotiate safe conduct for the Japanese through American lines, in exchange for the more than 250 internees being held by the Japanese. Two interpreters and four Japanese accompanied the two envoys as they moved through the crowd. Behind this group, Lieutenant Abiko, a man of whom the devil would have been proud, followed slowly but purposefully.

The American soldiers disarmed the four Japanese as Abiko moved forward. The GIs ordered Abiko to put his hands in the air, but instead of following orders, Abiko reached for a pouch slung over his shoulder. "American soldiers had long ago learned what that meant. The Japanese frequently carried on them a small hand grenade, which exploded on light contact and killed or seriously wounded everyone standing within a few yards. Japanese who had surrendered, would suddenly have one of these things in their hands and would commit suicide, taking several of their enemies with them by tapping the grenade either on the nearest enemy helmet or on their own." Hartendorp described what happened next: "As Abiko's hand reached his pouch, Major Gearheart in command of the tank unit grabbed a nearby carbine and shot him [Abiko] without even raising the gun to his shoulders."[6]

While Abiko lay writhing on the ground, the crowd of internees kicked and spit on him. They stripped the buttons and insignia from his uniform jacket as two internees grabbed hold of his feet and dragged him toward the emergency hospital in the main building lobby. On the way, several women burned him with cigarettes and two men slashed him with knives. Lt. Maude Denson Williams recorded the event in her book *To the Angels:* "I couldn't blame the people in the Plaza. . . . To us, this one man symbolized everything ugly and treacherous and vicious about the whole war. Recalling the faces of the old men in the Gym, the man who had lost 45 pounds in 30 days, the children searching the garbage cans for anything at all to eat, I could find no degree of pity for him."[7]

As American soldiers lifted Abiko to place him on a treatment table, a hand grenade rolled out of his hand onto the floor. It was picked up by a GI who placed it in his helmet and carried it outside.

Despite the feelings that Abiko engendered among the nurses and camp doctors, they gave him medical care. Dr. Stevenson looked at Abiko and back to Lieutenant Williams and said, "War makes animals of all of us." Williams described the following moments:

"I let go my breath and moved to help Dr. Stevenson, cutting away the Japanese uniform and looking up from the gaping wound in Abiko's abdomen to meet the doctor's eyes, not saying a word as I supported a broken arm until Shack [Lt. Shacklette] came with a splint. One of the Lieutenant's ears was nearly severed, and one cheek was gashed to the bone. Dr. Stevenson did the best he could, and when the bleeding was stopped, and the wounds dusted with sulfa and covered, he ordered Lieutenant Abiko put to bed in the next room. Four hours later Abiko was dead, and his body was removed to camp jail # 2, now being used as a morgue."[8]

All the internees were weak from malnutrition, and Dr. Stevenson and several of the nurses fainted that evening during the long, strenuous hours of caring for casualties. Their last meal had been a meager amount of moldy rice early that morning. The American soldiers willingly gave whatever food and K-rations they had to the internees and went without food for several days until supplies reached the camp. But people who were literally starving to death could eat only small amounts of food without vomiting. Lieutenant Ullom described how she and other nurses gradually took nourishment while caring for the newly wounded: "We took a cup of coffee and put a lot of powdered milk in it. About half a cup at a time would stay down. Our stomachs were so shrunk. The next day, we could tolerate about a cup."[9]

The American army was occupied with negotiations about the more than 50 Japanese who were holding approximately 160 men, 30 women, and several children as hostages in the education building. Finally, on 5 February, after hours of tense negotiating, terms were set. In exchange for the lives of the hostages, the Japanese soldiers would be escorted from camp by the American army and given safe conduct to the outskirts of Manila. At 0645 on 5 February the Japanese marched out of the education building. Internees lined both sides of the route as the Japanese were marched out of camp. Children called out, "Make them bow! Make them bow!" and adults hurled insults at the group. American troops left the Japanese at the edge of the city and returned to Santo Tomas. The freed Japanese entered Manila, where their soldiers and sailors were inflicting their own version of the rape of Nanking on innocent citizens. Although on a much smaller scale, the massacre of Manila was as savage and intense as that perpetrated in 1937 against the Chinese people; approximately one hundred thousand civilians were brutally killed. Once again the Japanese military lived up to its well-earned reputation as callous butchers.

General MacArthur came into camp on 5 February and was surrounded by grateful internees. The same day, two women internees obtained an American flag from a GI and unfurled it over the marquee on the main building. Internees gathered and sang "God Bless America" and the "Star Spangled Banner." Two men ran the flag up the pole by the main building and General MacArthur said, "Let no enemy ever take her down again!" The entire camp was moved to tears, laughter, and the celebration of freedom.

That afternoon, in yet another pointless display of brutality, the Japanese placed several of their large guns on the rooftops of buildings in Manila and shelled Santo Tomas. Lieutenant Young recorded the event: "All hell broke loose again. The Japanese started shelling our camp from the city. Many civilians killed and wounded. Our main bldg. being hit from the side. Fires broke out, water shortage, no where to sleep in safety, the gymnasium hit by a shell with casualties among the patients. Dorm captain wounded, probably unable to see again. In other words, we are on the front lines again and nowhere for us to go."[10]

On the same day Bilibid was liberated by the First Cavalry, Thirty-seventh Division, and the Fourty-forth Tank Battalion. That liberation followed a terrifying battle in which the POWs and internees might well have been killed. Lt. Beatrice Chambers gives us an insider's view: "I heard them coming in. I went on top of the wall of Bilibid, upstairs. I crouched behind the wall there and watched the tanks. I was never so happy in my life. You see the Gestapo [Japanese Kempeitai] had a place right opposite this Bilibid Prison. They were horrible, I mean just like the German Gestapo, the Japanese Gestapo. . . . They [a U.S. tank] came up to this house where the Gestapo was and he threw that liquid fire. Man, I was never so happy to see that go down, it just folded up like worms."[11]

The prisoners from Bilibid were taken to Santo Tomas within two days of their rescue. Santo Tomas was in foul shape as a result of overcrowding, Japanese shelling, and lack of sanitation facilities. Lieutenant Chambers joined the other former POW army nurses in treating wounded American soldiers and internees in a camp still under attack, in a city still at war. As she told it: "All the lights were knocked out. All the toilets were knocked out [would not flush]. I got in line because I had to go to the toilet. Well, I got out of the line, and I sat on a stairway between these two great huge pillars. . . . I'll be damn if a mortar shell didn't come and get everybody in that line I was in. I had the shakes afterwards. I no sooner moved, two minutes, one minute, and this mortar came in."[12]

Seeing people wounded and killed in battle was bad enough, but watching innocent civilians and former POWs fired on out of spite was almost too much for the nurses to endure. Lieutenant Chambers expressed the feelings of all medical personnel: "We had terrible casualties. The poor prisoners . . . they were killed or maimed. There was one beautiful girl, only 17, I'll never forget her. Half her face was taken off."[13]

On 7 February the Japanese shelled Santo Tomas again. A shell hit the main building, killing several internees and wounding others. Lt. Denny Williams recalled: "I remember Mrs. Foley particularly. Her husband was killed when the shell hit their room, and she lost one of her arms at the shoulder. She was brought to the emergency hospital and her teen-age daughter, Mary Frances, came with her. Mrs. Foley kept asking about her husband and fifteen year old Mary Frances told her he was fine. She knew he was dead, but she did not want to tell her mother when she was facing surgery for her amputated arm. Kids grew up fast in Santo Tomas. . . . It was heartbreaking to see people killed and injured after they had endured more than three years of Japanese captivity. It was just heartbreaking."[14]

On 9 February one hundred Army nurses, led by the chief nurse, Lt. Col. Nola Forrest, and forty army doctors arrived from Leyte to care for the sick and wounded. They received a warm welcome from POW nurses and internees alike.

On 10 February heavy shelling hit the camp again, this time falling on the hospital on the second floor of the education building. The following day, the more than 165 patients in the education building hospital were moved to the Quezon Institute by ambulance and truck. In the next week, several hundred more patients were transported to the institute. In all, the shelling after the camp's liberation killed seventeen internees and injured more than ninety, including Lt. Vivian Weissblatt, a forty-year-old civilian dietitian who was commissioned by the army after the war began.

On the same day, in the midst of shell fire, Lt. Bertha Dworsky and John Henderson were married in the museum of the main building. Lieutenant Young remarked on the wedding: "A few days ago we couldn't have thrown rice at them," she said. "We needed it too badly to eat, but to-nite we could throw all we wanted."[15] The following night Lt. Alice Hahn and Eddie Powers pronounced their marriage vows in the same museum.

Living conditions inside the camp were growing steadily worse. Most people in the main building had moved to its far side to get away from the shelling and were sleeping on the floor. Water was scarce, toilets could not be flushed, and most of the camp population was sick from overeating.[16]

On the morning of 12 February, the POW nurses, the army dietitians, and an army physiotherapist were notified that they would be leaving in ten minutes and could bring only their musette bags. The nurses were loaded onto open trucks and driven to Dewey Boulevard, one of Manila's main thoroughfares, where a plane waited to carry them to Leyte. Japanese gunfire buzzed around the aircraft as they taxied and made their ascent. Lt. Helen Cassiani remembered: "I can see them now. The pilot said, 'Now girls, move up front.' We literally were piled one on the other, four or five deep. 'Let's free that tail, free that tail,' and of course he's off. I felt sure that damn tail would never let go of that blacktop. But we made it. We cleared the power lines and everything."[17]

Not long after leaving Manila, the C-47 developed engine trouble and made an unscheduled landing on Mindoro, an American-held island in the Philippines, south of Luzon. Someone decided that an air crash would be particularly disastrous, so the nurses were divided into two groups and continued the trip on separate planes. When they reached Leyte, the nurses were admitted to the 126th General Hospital. Seventeen of the group were ill enough to require intravenous fluids and were admitted to a hospital building. The others were housed in hospital tents along the beach.

During their eight-day stay on the island, each nurse received a complete physical examination, followed by plenty of relaxation and sleep. Army Class A uniforms were flown in from Australia, and each nurse was promoted one grade. At a special ceremony, General Guy Denitt presented each former POW with a Presidential Citation and a bronze star with two oak leaf clusters. Lts. Rosemary Hogan, Rita Palmer, and Frances Nash received the Purple Heart for wounds inflicted before surrendering to the Japanese. Lt. Mary B. Brown Menzie was awarded the Purple Heart for wounds received while a prisoner of war, and Lt. Vivian Weissblatt received the Purple Heart for wounds received during the Japanese shelling of Santo Tomas.[18] On 20 February 1945 the former POW army nurses left Leyte for the United States. Eleven were still ill enough to be flown aboard a hospital plane. The remaining fifty-six were split into groups and traveled aboard two C-54Es. The plush planes had been sent to Leyte with the sole purpose of bringing the former POW nurses home. The trip would take at least twenty-four hours flying time, not counting the hours spent on the ground for servicing the aircraft and feeding the crew and passengers. Lt. Eunice Young recalled their first stop on Saipan: "We were welcomed with open arms and [we] couldn't keep the tears back when we had a large Coke with [the message] 'Win for Liberty' on it."[19] Lt. Madeline Ullom remembered what a luxury it was to ride in the C-54E: "Each of us got a whole seat to sleep on. With the armrest up, it was the best bed we'd had in more than three years. We didn't do much talking on the way back to the States. We were all so exhausted that we slept most of the way."[20]

When the nurses arrived at Hickam Field in Honolulu, they deplaned to the music of an army band playing the "Star Spangled Banner" and knelt to kiss the ground. The group was billeted at the nurses' quarters and served steak with all the trimmings. Lt. Bertha Dworsky Henderson recalled that time: "We had tub baths, and we had a permanent. Somebody even found some silk stockings for us."[21]

The nurses remained in Honolulu for two nights, then continued their journey. They arrived in San Francisco on 24 February, where their planes landed simultaneously at Hamilton Air Field. Following a welcoming ceremony the former POWs were admitted to Letterman General Hospital, where they received further physical examinations and medical tests.

On 21 February 1945, while the army nurses continued their journey homeward and the navy nurses were still prisoners of war in Los Baños Internment Camp, the decapitated bodies of Carroll Grinnell, A.F. Duggleby, E.E. Johnson, and Clifford Larsen were found buried near Harrison Park in Manila. On 23 February 1945, a memorial service was held for these four men.

At Los Baños the cruel treatment of the Japanese continued to take its toll on the internees. On 28 January 1945 a particularly heinous incident occurred that was deeply engraved into the minds of the navy nurses. Although fruit trees grew just outside the camp fence, the Japanese had forbidden the internees to pick the fruit. One male internee, George Louis, scaled the fence in an attempt to bring fruit to several of the pregnant women prisoners. As he was returning to camp with the fruit, Japanese sentries shot him without warning him to halt. "Mr. Louis was dragged inside the fence and left on the ground, bleeding . . . so the prisoners could watch him die," Lieutenant Todd said. "We weren't allowed to help him. He was a very proud man . . . he didn't cry out."[22]

The Japanese insisted that Louis, who was still alive, must be executed immediately because sentries were ordered to shoot to kill. Members of the Internee Committee and fellow prisoners asked permission to take Louis to the camp hospital so he could be treated. Moments later, a single shot was heard and the Internee Committee requested the body for burial. Although the Japanese insisted that Louis had been killed by a single gunshot as he reentered the camp, the camp medical director, Dr. Dana Nance, stated in his official report: "The body had been pierced by two bullets. One bullet had a wound of entrance above the outer border of the right clavicle (collar bone) and an exit wound along the upper border of the corresponding scapula. This missile grazed the scapula but struck no vital organs—did not even enter the chest cavity—and was in no sense a mortal wound. The other bullet entered the skull in the right frontal region and blew his brains out in the left occipital region. It would appear that this man was executed or given the coup de grace after having sustained minor injury."[23] The Internee Committee filed a formal protest.

News that the other camps in and around Manila had been freed made its way to Los Baños. The Japanese set up machine guns encircling the camp, barrels facing inward. On 22 February 1945 a Japanese soldier arrived at Los Baños with a message for the commandant, "Kill the prisoners." Lt. Edwina Todd remembered that day: "At that time the Japanese had only 200 guards at Los Banos. And fortunately for us, our commander was a very conservative man and decided to wait until morning and until his some 8,000 troops came back into camp to do the job."[24] Throughout that night, the machine guns remained silent, but their presence was a terrifying reminder to the prisoners that their deaths could be imminent.

At dawn on 23 February 1945, while the Japanese did their daily calisthenics, a meticulously timed combined operation to liberate Los Baños began. The operation, choreographed as intricately as a ballet, involved many components working toward a single purpose. Its participants included Filipino guerrillas, the Eleventh Airborne, the 127th Airborne Engineering Battalion, Recon Platoons

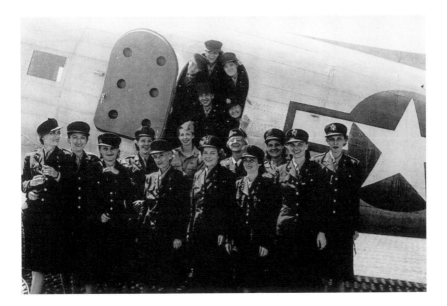

A group of Army nurses pose before leaving Leyte for Hawaii. There were not enough brass hat devices to complete their newly issued uniforms; U.S. Army Signal Corps.

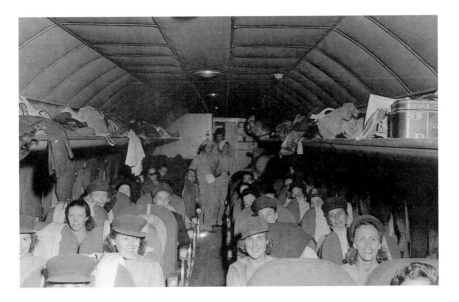

Freed U.S. Army nurses aboard one of the planes that carried their group from Leyte to Hawaii; U.S. Army Signal Corps.

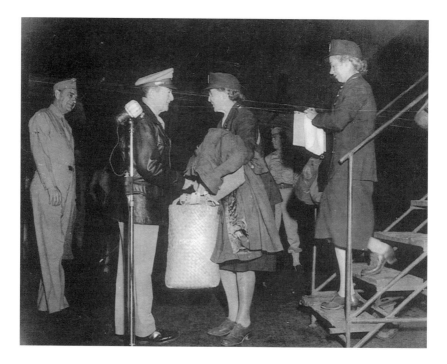

Lt. Gen. Robert Richardson Jr., Commanding General USAFPOA, greets Capt. Josephine Nesbit, ANC, as she steps from the plane in Hawaii on 21 February 1945; U.S. Army Signal Corps.

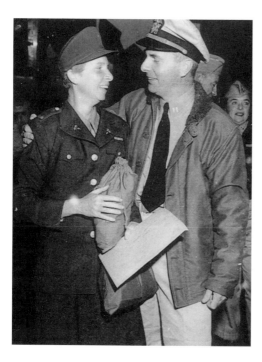

1st Lt. Beatrice Chambers greeted by her brother, Lt. James Chambers, USNR, after she arrived in Honolulu; U.S. Army Signal Corps.

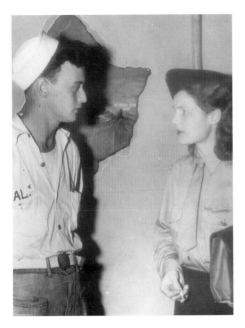

At a stopover on Guam, navy nurse Lt. Mary R. Harrington (wearing an Army Nurse Corps uniform) chats with a sailor from her hometown in South Dakota; U.S. Navy photograph.

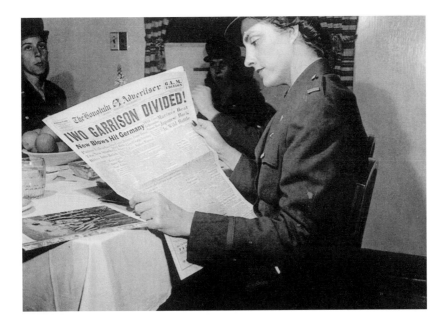

1st Lt. Earlyn M. Black, ANC, repatriated from Santo Tomas Internment Camp, reads her first newspaper in over three years upon her recent arrival in the Hawaiian Islands; U.S. Army Signal Corps.

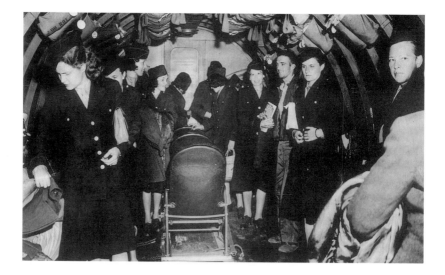

Navy nurses prepare to leave plane after arriving in Hawaii. The nurses are wearing Army Nurse Corps uniforms because no Navy Nurse Corps uniforms were available at any station prior to Honolulu; U.S. Navy photograph.

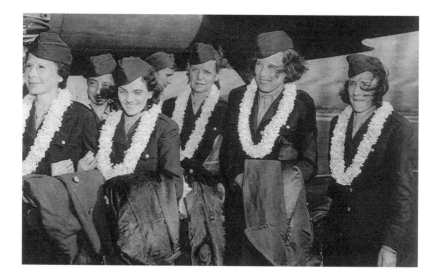

Navy nurses after deplaning at Pearl Harbor, Hawaii, on their way to the U.S. (Left to right): Chief nurse Lt. Comdr. Laura Cobb, Lts. Margaret Nash, Goldia O'Haver, Bertha Evans, Helen Gorzelanski; U.S. Navy photograph.

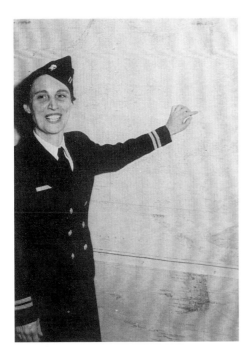

Lt. Leona Jackson pointing at a map showing Guam, where she was captured by the Japanese three years earlier. She later returned to Guam as senior navy nurse in 1945; U.S. Navy photograph.

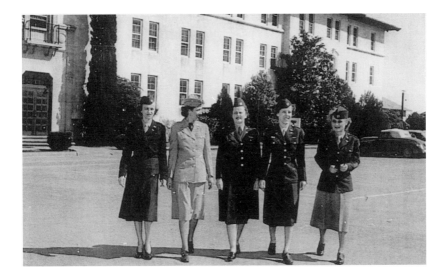

In March 1949 five former POW nurses attended the Hospital Administration Course at Medical Field Services School, Brooke Army Medical Center, Fort Sam Houston, Texas. (Left to right): Capts. Mary Jean Reppak, Ruth Stoltz, Helen Hennessey, Eunice Young, and Eula Fails; U.S. Army Signal Corps.

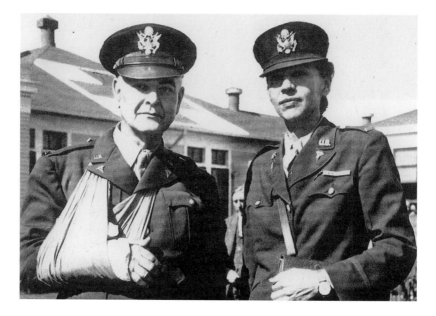

Col. J.W. Duckworth and 1st Lt. Frances L. Nash are reunited at Letterman General Hospital in San Francisco, February 1945; authors' archives.

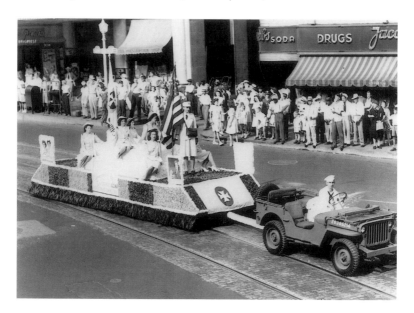

1945 homecoming parade and bond drive: Georgia welcomed 1st Lt. Frances L. Nash (standing on float); authors' archives.

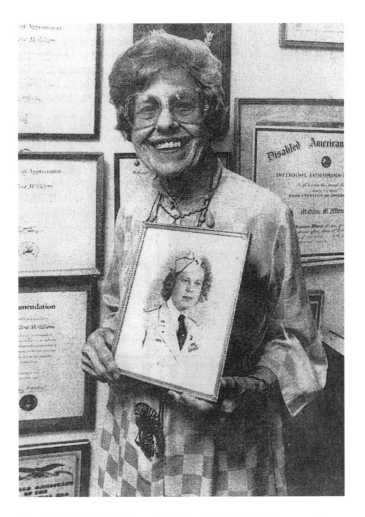

Lt. Col. Madeline Ullom, ANC (Ret.), 1989, holding a post-World War II photograph of herself in uniform; authors' archives.

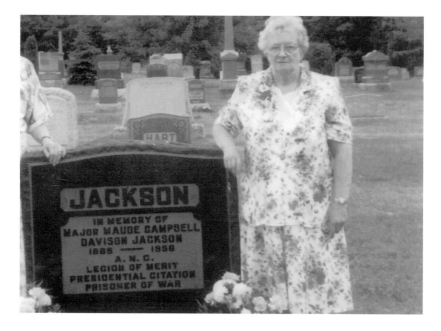

Mrs. Velma Campbell Willis, niece of Major Maude Campbell Davison Jackson, standing beside the Major's tombstone prior to Cannington, Ontario's celebration of "Major Maude Day" on 1 July 1992; authors' archives.

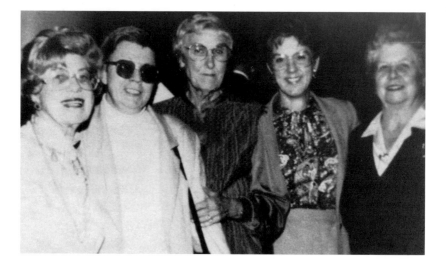

Three former POWs with authors in 1989. (Left to right): Lt. Col. Madeline Ullom, ANC (Ret.); Evelyn Monahan; Lt. Col. Hattie R. Brantley, ANC (Ret.); Rosemary Neidel-Greenlee; Helen Cassiani Nestor; authors' archives.

of the Eleventh Airborne, the 511th Parachute Infantry Regimental Combat Team, the 188th Parachute Infantry Regimental Combat Team, and the 672d Amphibian Tractor Battalion. The operation hinged on split-second timing and cooperation among the various units. Guerrillas attacked and killed Japanese sentries minutes before paratroopers jumped from nine C-47s in sight of the camp, and amphtracks of the 672d made their way across Laguna de Bay and inland to Los Baños.

The internees had been without food for the last two days and fully expected to be machine-gunned by the Japanese in a matter of hours. Lt. Edwina Todd was standing in her barracks doorway looking up at the sky as daylight crept into Los Baños. She described those pivotal moments: "I saw a little white patch floating down, surely a parachute—a parachute dropping food," she thought. Soon many parachutes were falling toward earth, and as the nine planes flew in formation, Todd could read the word "Rescue" painted on their sides. Tears were streaming down her face just when she thought she could no longer cry. The nurse standing next to her, an avowed atheist, was praying in a loud voice, "Dear God, don't let them get shot, dear God, don't let them get shot," over and over. In minutes, American tanks crashed through the camp walls. The soldiers were being treated with atabrine for malaria, and their complexions were jaundiced as a result. Many of the internees were hysterical because they mistook the soldiers riding on the tanks for Japanese. Not until the Americans leaped from the tanks and people could see how tall and large they were did the internees feel secure. "How big they seemed, like Supermen."[25]

After killing the Japanese soldiers present, American troops had to move the 2,157 internees out of Los Baños across Laguna de Bay and into Manila. To facilitate a rapid evacuation, they set fire to the straw barracks to prevent internees from returning to them. Although the 253 Japanese guards were dead, speed was essential. Approximately 8,000 Japanese troops were stationed only eight miles away, and the rescuers numbered fewer than 500. Several of the navy nurses pushed carts bearing their meager possessions and bandages. Lt. Susie Pitcher was so swollen with beriberi that she could barely walk.[26]

The evacuation went more smoothly than Lt. Col. Walsh and the men of the Eleventh Airborne Division had anticipated. The chief nurse, Laura Cobb, directed the loading of the sickest patients and one current casualty onto the amphtracs. Many internees who had been immobile for months got up and walked. As a long line of evacuees neared Laguna de Bay, Japanese snipers fired on them. Nurses and civilians threw themselves to the ground, and Lts. Edwina Todd and Margaret Nash placed their bodies over the three-day-old and one-week-old infants they were carrying; the babies survived unhurt. The gunfire continued as amphtracs carried the internees across the lake to waiting ambulances and trucks that would take them to Manila. Upon their arrival at Bilibid Prison, navy nurses set up a hospital ward for the women and children rescued from Los Baños.

Ten days later the nurses were relieved of duty by army nurses and flown to Leyte. Edwina Todd recalled that they flew by C-47 to Leyte, where army nurses gave them army uniforms and silk stockings. From Leyte they flew in Admiral Thomas C. Kinkaid's plane to Samar and via Guam, Kwajalein, and the Johnston Islands to Pearl Harbor, where they spent two days. While at the Navy Hospital Aiea Heights, they were reintroduced to cosmetics, hot baths, and beauty parlors. The women were most delighted to meet other navy nurses for the first time since their imprisonment and to exchange their borrowed army clothing for navy uniforms.[27]

As was true of all the former POW nurses, the three years they spent as captives of the Japanese marked their physical appearance. "Lt. Cmdr. Susan J. English, with a Naval hospital here, said she was unable to recognize some of the interned nurses she had known best. 'They've aged 10 years, when they should have aged three.'"[28]

On 10 March 1945 the eleven navy nurses arrived in San Francisco aboard a navy transport plane and were admitted to the Oakland Naval Hospital, where they were examined and treated for the next several weeks.

Individual hometowns welcomed the nurses home. Typical was

the welcome extended to Margaret Nash, by her hometown of
Wilkes-Barre, Pennsylvania and reported on by her hometown
newspaper. Twenty-five thousand people lined the route to her
home to greet her.

More than 5,000 assembled at the Lehigh Valley Railroad station yesterday afternoon to greet Lieutenant
Nash. When she stepped from the train she was met by
members of her family and then John J. McSweeney,
chairman of the reception committee of the Lee Park
Honor Roll and Civic Corporation extended formal
greetings in behalf of the community. She was escorted
to an open car provided by Andrew Sordoni where the
official ceremonies were held. While making her way
along the platform, a stranger thrust an envelope into her
hand. Later it developed that there was a Miraculous
Medal inside. Nurses and nurses' aides from Mercy
Hospital, her alma mater, formed a guard of honor. She
received from the hospital a bouquet of roses. . . . Mayor
Con McCole presented the key to the city . . . at hometown ceremonies.
   At Sullivan and South Main streets, Miss Nash's car
was halted while members of the 12th Ward Club pre-
sented her with flowers. The P.O.S. of A. also presented a
bouquet.
   When the procession arrived at Barney and Hanover
Streets, Miss Nash's car was driven to nearby Mercy
Hospital where [she] was greeted by a group of nuns.
   At St. Aloysius' Church, several thousand parishioners
were waiting for her. Escorted by Mr. McSweeney, Miss
Nash went into the church between a guard of honor,
consisting of St. Aloysius' Boy Scouts. She was met by the
Rev. Gerard Canican and the Rev. Francis Durkin, who
accompanied Miss Nash to the altar where the party knelt
in a prayer of thanksgiving. Members of the congregation
joined them and stood as the party filed from the church.
   It was while she was leaving the church that Miss Nash

gave way the first time to emotion. She wiped the tears from her eyes repeatedly.

"It was only prayer that sustained me," she commented.

As the procession headed for Oxford Street and home, Miss Nash expressed concern about her mother.

"I hope she is not left alone," she said, looking at the milling thousands along the way. She was assured her mother did not lack for company.

A few minutes later, the dramatic moment of the whole trip arrived when Lieutenant Nash, standing in the moving car, sighted her mother on the porch.

"Mother! Mother!" she exclaimed with outstretched arms and tears rolling down her cheeks. It was only a matter of seconds until she was in her mother's arms. The journey half way around the world was ended.[29]

The welcome Nash received was owed to every man and woman in uniform. This fact is reflected in the following comments:

"Members of the armed forces, wherever they may be serving, will take heart at the welcome accorded Miss Nash. This is how America regards its defenders, although it does not often have the opportunity to show its true feelings. The Lee Park girl symbolized the hardships and sacrifices of thousands, now serving their country, and no one can have the least doubt in the future of this anthracite community's appreciation. Miss Nash unwittingly has performed another service in buoying up the spirits of countless young men and women in uniform who may have been speculating about how the home folks felt. They know today."[30]

About two weeks following their return to the United States, the army nurses who were well enough were granted sixty-day leaves and were allowed to extend them to ninety days if they felt they needed more time. Most of the army nurses and dietitians headed for their homes and families. For the first time in more than three years, they were free and on their own. The group that had counted on each other for survival would now be scattered to various states and hometowns, where they would face the task of reacclimating to a free world as individuals. They had shared a unique experience. Few with whom they spoke outside their group would truly understand the price they had paid for the freedom of all Americans. They had passed into the annals of history, but it would be decades before their story would reach the pages of history.

11

Home at Last

All months are special—but March 3, 1945, more so to me. Being back in my beloved Georgia, all feeling safe with Daddy and Mother, after a nightmare of threats, horrible experiences and such needless starvation, brutal killings, needless suffering, being forced to look on as they tortured the native Filipino work animal, the carabaos. I don't hate anyone, but in my heart, I will never forget.

Lt. Frances L. Nash, ANC

The world had changed in many ways during the more than thirty-seven months the nurses had spent in a war zone and as prisoners of war of the Japanese. They learned how close they had come to being killed by their captors. The liberation of Santo Tomas seemed even more miraculous when the nurses learned that the Japanese had planned to kill all the inhabitants of the camp. General MacArthur's orders to the First Cavalry and the Forty-fourth Tank Division to fight their way straight to Santo Tomas more than likely saved the lives of the POWs. Lt. Minnie Breese commented on their narrow escape: "They had gasoline tanks underneath the main stairway, and they were going to burn us all to death. That's the reason they locked us in there, but they didn't get around to it. They [Americans] came in too quick. They didn't get around to lighting the fire."[1]

The towns and cities they had left when they went to the peacetime Philippines had been changed radically by the world war that had overtaken them far from home, surrounded them with the Battles of Bataan and Corregidor, seen them held by the Japanese as prisoners of war, engulfed them in the Japanese shelling of Santo Tomas, and finally saw them make their way home through war-torn skies. Thousands were busy at work in defense plants, thousands more on armed forces military installations around the country.

The nurses had returned home, but home had changed forever. Many found that relatives they had left behind were no longer waiting for their return. Some brothers and sisters were serving their country in foreign theaters of war. Some parents were no longer living, and many had lost friends on battlefields. Lt. Helen Cassiani was heartbroken when she returned to the reality of her mother's death and faced new feelings connected to her imprisonment. She had joined the Army Nurse Corps a naive twenty-four-year-old and returned four years later, fifty-nine pounds lighter and considerably more mature and with her priorities reordered. "I believe that bad things as well as good things help to mold whatever you become, so I never was bitter about the experience. The only thing I was ever bitter about was the fact that more information, more definite information couldn't have been available to our families. I had left a sick mother. My father had been dead many years. I think the only notice they [she] had was a postcard-type notice from the War Department. 'Your daughter stationed in the Philippines is missing in action.' For almost a year and a half, that's all they knew. . . . The next communication was, 'Your daughter is a prisoner of war of the Japanese and she is imprisoned in Santo Tomas.' They did say what prison camp I was in and for any further information to contact the Red Cross," Cassiani said. "My mother died, had another heart attack, three days before my liberation. So if I'm sad, and bitter about anything, I feel that my experience and the treatment of that experience [lack of communication with families] very likely contributed to another heart attack, and her death. The fact that my mother died three days before my liberation. This hurt me, you know, very much. So much that, yes, indeed for quite a few years, I would have one dream, a recurring dream. Not every night, you understand. But, when I would have it, it was always exactly the same, and it had to do with my mother . . . I could see my mother in the dream, but she gave no sign that she recognized me. It was very hard."[2]

A few learned of a parent's death while they were still in Santo Tomas, but the knowledge came to them long after the fact, and they had to deal with the reality when they returned. Lieutenant Brantley put it thus: "It's strange to learn that someone you've thought of all along as alive has actually been dead two years. It really let you know just how cut off from the world you were. Made you feel kind of powerless."[3]

Several of the former POW army nurses had to deal with the death of a POW fiancé or husband. Others had to live with not knowing where their POW husbands or fiancés were, or whether they were alive or long dead. For Lt. Denny Williams, the news she learned soon after her return was not good. Her husband, Lt. William R. Williams, Thirty-first Infantry, United States Army, was killed on 9 January 1945, when the *Encura Maru*, a Japanese POW ship taking American POWs to Tokyo, was hit and sunk by U.S. bombers in the harbor of Takao, Formosa.

Lt. Minnie Breese Stubbs did not learn what had become of her fiancé until late October 1945. She recalled the memory years later: "He was sent to Japan and he didn't get out until they dropped the atom bomb. . . . In fact, he saw the atom bomb and didn't know what it was. He was stationed [imprisoned] in Nagasaki. I didn't know he was alive until I was back on duty at Percy Jones and he called me from San Francisco in September, or October [October]. He came back on a slow boat because he was tired and he didn't want to fly back. He was liberated in September. But he was commandant of the camp and so he had to stay and turn it over and all that. So then he took a boat back as he was sick. He had schistosomiasis. So they shipped him to Walter Reed where he stayed for a year and a half."[4]

Readjustment to life for the former POW nurses was far from easy. Habits learned to help one survive the camp were not easy to drop. Nurses found themselves hiding things and saving food that might have meant the difference between life and death in Santo Tomas. At times, not even a sympathetic parent fully understood their actions. According to Lt. Frances Nash: "Even now, here at my parents' peaceful farm in Wilkes County, I am hiding things from the Japs. After nearly three years of concealing every rag, every piece of string from my captors, I just cannot feel safe in leaving anything I own right out on my dressing table. The other day I found myself slipping an important letter under the mattress. Thank heavens my mother didn't see that, it might have hurt her feelings, just as the steak episode did." Nash went on to describe this incident: "The abundance of food here in the States still amazes me. At dinner the other night we had steak, more steak than I could eat, and I carefully cut off half the meat and asked mother to put it away for the following day. 'Put it away! Why go ahead and eat it, there's plenty more,' she explained, hurt because I didn't think there was any more in the kitchen. When you've eaten boiled canna lily roots, you have a tendency to think about the next meal."[5]

Many of the former POWs were balanced on the edge of wanting contact and appreciating people who wanted to honor them and needing quiet and hoping for time where no questions were asked and no answers were expected. For many, military leave at home meant a whirlwind of speeches, dinners at the local Grange or Kiwanis Club, and a constant stream of visiting relatives and friends. As wonderful as it was to be home and honored, these women were still feeling the effects of malnutrition, illnesses, and emotional stress. Decades later, the Veterans Administration and others finally came to recognize that military nurses in combat conditions experience post-traumatic stress disorder (PTSD). Many of the military nurses who had been prisoners of war died before this fact was acknowledged, but several of the former POWs have since been diagnosed as having PTSD as a result of their World War II experiences.

After ninety days of leave at home, the former POWs reported to redistribution centers of their choosing for reassignment. Each woman was told she could pick her next duty station after she com-

pleted her time at the redistribution center. The centers were located in Atlantic City, New Jersey; Asheville, North Carolina; Mi-
ami, Florida; Santa Barbara, California; and Lake Placid, New York.
Lt. Madeline Ullom spoke of her time at a center, obviously a pleasant memory: "We were supposed to stay at least two weeks, but
could stay longer if we wanted to. I went to the Lake Placid Club,
which was 'ultra.' I had the bridal suite. It had a porch on one end
that was glassed in, and then the one on the west side was open.
You could engage in sports, skiing, riding or boating, or anything
you wanted. I used to play cards at the women's club. Somebody
was inviting you all the time for lunch or dinner."[6]

Between recreation and meals, the redistribution centers were
busy testing and reclassifying troops from the European and Mediterranean theaters of war for discharge or reassignment. Reassign-
ments were usually for the Far East because the country was gearing
up for an all-out assault on Japan. The former POW nurses were
not considered for reassignment in the Pacific but were asked their
preference for their next assignment. Whenever possible, their re-
quests were granted. Many of the nurses picked hospitals in the
South because they had become accustomed to hot weather. Later
Lieutenant Ullom volunteered for a research project at Fort Bevins,
Massachusetts, to study clothing for cold and wet climates. For two
weeks the group camped on the ground at the top of Mount Washington and hiked all over the mountains of New Hampshire. They
slept on the ground in sleeping bags and for the first time were
fitted with combat boots made for a woman's foot.[7]

Former POWs were frequently asked to go on bond tours to
raise money. After hiking through the New Hampshire mountains
on the cold weather project, Ullom was assigned to a bond tour.
The first stop on that assignment was Fort Lee, Virginia, where she
and five others learned public speaking. Following that course,
Ullom was sent on a bond tour of Alabama. She spent six weeks in
Montgomery, a week in Mobile, a week in Birmingham, and a week
in Tuscaloosa. "Those people down south, they did ferry you
around. It was really fun. They'd meet you at the train; you'd have
roses in your room at the hotel, and they took you all over," she

said. "We'd talk on the radio at 6:00 in the morning, to the school kids at nine, then the Women's Club, and then the Kiwanis and Lion's Clubs at noon. I was on the rubber chicken circuit. In the afternoon, it was back to the women's clubs, because women down south played cards and had lots of clubs. At night we'd have rallies and dinners and banquets. We got grades on making a quota."[8]

Of all the cities and towns in Alabama that Ullom visited, the one that stood out in her mind was Jasper. As she had for so many things in her life, she volunteered for the trip.

Once they said to me, "Now you haven't been to Jasper, and you don't have to go to Jasper. You don't have to but they have a lot of money in Jasper, and they'll buy a lot of bonds."

"Well," I said, "let me go to Jasper."

They said, "Now Jasper is different. It's not like Montgomery, it's not like Mobile or any of those other places."

"Oh," I said, "I don't care. I want to go to Jasper."

Well I got off the train at Jasper. I tell you there was nobody there to meet me. So, I took my suitcase and I started down the road. It wasn't much of a road. It was a mining town, a coal mining town. Finally, I saw somebody, so I asked where Mr. Gardner was, if he knew him. He said, "Yes." So I asked, where I could find him. He stuck his thumb up and said, "Over there." I started down to "over there." I got to this building and I opened the door. It was a store. I asked if Mr. Gardner was there.

"Yes."

"Well where is he?"

"In there."

So I went "in there" and here he was sitting with his feet on the rim of a pot bellied stove, doing the ledger. There was a window pane and it was full of people looking in the window at me. They bought a lot of bonds in Jasper, and they did all right.[9]

Several of the nurses went on recruiting drives for the Army

Nurse Corps. Lt. Rita Palmer and one other nurse were sent to New York for eighteen days. After more than three years as POWs, they could find fun in almost anything, but that New York trip seemed extra special. Palmer remembered the experience: "We had a ball going to plays and painting our fingernails, and going to Elizabeth Arden's and getting all gussied up. We had a wonderful time."[10]

All of the former POW nurses had a lot to catch up on in their personal and professional lives. Many of them read old magazines such as *Life, Look, Time,* and *Newsweek* in an effort to fill in a wide knowledge gap in general events and war news. Some asked to be placed on the wards in military hospitals so they could educate themselves on new medications, techniques, and treatments. After several months, most were promoted to head nurse positions or went on to other assignments.

Several of the group were looking forward to returning to civilian life as soon as possible after the war was over. The general rule for length of service was "for the duration plus ninety days." Lt. Bertha Dworsky Henderson expressed the feelings of those counting the days until their discharge: "We were not allowed to go back overseas. So, I chose to go to Fort Lawton in Seattle, Washington. I was sent there in July of '45. In the meantime my husband had come to the States. He came to Texas and then went up to Seattle with me. I was stationed there, but I knew that I didn't want to continue in the Army much longer. Only just as long as I had to, to get established in civilian life. So I got out of the Army in 1946. I just sort of tried to meld into civilian life and be a homemaker and a mother."[11]

Madeline Ullom and sixteen other army nurses decided to make a career of the military, and some spent up to thirty years in the Nurse Corps of the U.S. Army, the U.S. Navy, or U.S. Air Force, the latter established in 1947. One of the former POW navy nurses, Lt. W. Leona Jackson, became the director of the Navy Nurse Corps in 1954.[12]

America was anxious to return to the conditions that existed before her entrance into World War II. Women were fired from their defense plant jobs and expected to put making a home and raising a family at the top of their agendas. America no longer needed women working outside the home. Millions of returning servicemen would need civilian jobs, and the country was focused on that objective. There was a silent consensus that the country would forget what women can and did endure and remember them as the "return to normalcy" demanded: domestic, safe, and fragile. The emergency had subsided and, with it, the need to "place women in harm's way." Combat veterans were men. No woman had earned the Combat Infantry Badge, and history would focus on those who had earned that distinction. Women would be remembered as having safe jobs behind the lines. Even members of the subsequent Army and Navy Nurse Corps were not regularly taught the history of their predecessors' services in World War II, and the former POWs had signed statements agreeing not to speak of the atrocities they had seen. In an undeclared "conspiracy of silence," being a POW was presented to the nurses as a stigma, something to be hidden, even from their own families. At the redistribution centers and reorientation programs, army nurses were told that military nurses needed to become "ladies" again. Lt. Col. Hattie R. Brantley remembered that instruction and its long-lasting effects. "You didn't talk about sex, you didn't talk about having been a prison of war. When we came home, so help me, we had what they called 'reorientation' in Little Rock, Arkansas. I was assigned to go there and be debriefed. As sure as I'm standing here, that guy stood up there and said, 'Now you're going off to your assignments and whatever you do, just keep it [combat and POW experiences] to yourself, don't talk about it.' They absolutely told us that. They treated it as if it was a stigma. And of course, we didn't *care* to talk about it in those days. I never talked to my family about it. I never talked to anybody about it. It was just one of those things."[13]

These army and navy nurses quietly faded out of the history they had lived. Soon, no one except those who had lived the history first-hand would remember that army and navy nurses had cared for the wounded in Manila, Bataan, and Corregidor. The memory of military women at the battles that during World War II were synonymous with the Alamo was neglected and not told to those who followed in their footsteps. America lost a national treasure, and American heroines who had risked all for freedom were banished from the written history they had helped to write. History books on World War II would rarely mention nurses in combat zones, and less frequently, do they broach the topic of military women as prisoners of war.

Perhaps it is time that our nation's history books tell the stories of military women, of former POW army and navy nurses who were willing to pay the ultimate price for freedom. Like Queen Esther in the Old Testament, each can be said to have answered her country's need with the words, "I go, and if I perish, I perish." These women have stood the test of patriotism and have actively helped to pass on the gift of freedom to all of us who enjoy it now. As former POW navy nurse W. Leona Jackson said in a speech given in 1942 following her repatriation as a Japanese prisoner of war: "Whatever the cost, it is worth it. The price we pay is a legacy which we hand down to generations yet to come."[14]

Appendix A

Tribute to
Major Maude C. Davison, ANC

If ever a group needed a leader with sterling characteristics, it was when the Japanese took us captive on 6 May 1942 at Fort Mills, Corregidor. Captain Maude C. Davison was superbly qualified. She was well educated and had long years of military service. If this were to be our lot, we were very fortunate to be recipients of her wisdom. I was stationed with her at Sternberg General Hospital in Manila where she was Chief Nurse of the hospital and Chief Nurse for the Department of the Philippines U.S. Army.

Once at Santo Tomas Internment Camp, she was ill. Ann Mealer asked me to special her. She was an ideal patient. Uppermost in her mind was to rapidly recover so she could assume her duties in the nurses' interests and patients' nursing care.

She was alert, observant and detailed from the smallest to the largest problems. She analyzed fully, planned comprehensively, organized completely and implemented smoothly. She ever sought available solutions and after considerations, she always selected the best. She made decisions instantly or over a period of time when indicated. A retinue of very high ranking Japanese officers attempted to enter the nurses' quarters. A Japanese attempted to pull the sheet covering the entrance. She was immediately on her feet as she demanded, "Halt! You cannot come in here without permission." Discussions which involved placement and duties of nurses were very long. She worked well with Japanese Commandants and the Executive Committee and others at Santo Tomas Internment Camp. In final analysis, the military nurses were kept as a unit. She was given the title "Superintendent of Nurses" for the 150 bed hospital, 80 bed isolation hospital: Main Building, Hospital and Children's Clinics.

On Bataan and Corregidor the military called us "Angels." The name persisted. In 1983 we were presented with plaques which read:

"Is commended for distinguished service and unswerving devotion to duty during the period December 1941 to February 1945. You served with honor and endured indescribable hardships and incredible physical, psychological and professional challenges with a courage above and beyond the call of duty. Through these noble deeds you became the role model of Army Nursing in upholding the finest traditions of the Army Nurse Corps, the Army Medical Department and the United States Army. Bernhard T. Mittemsy, Lieutenant General, The Surgeon General."

If this were for us, you can imagine the weight of responsibility for the nurses and nursing care in Santo Tomas and the battlefields, carried by Captain Maude C. Davison.

Madeline M. Ullom, Lt. Col., USA, NC (Ret.) N123
29 October 1991

Appendix B

Pre-World War II Duty Stations of U.S. Navy Nurses Held as POWs by the Japanese

U.S. Naval Hospital at Canacao, Luzon, Philippine Islands:*

Chief Nurse Lt.(jg) Cobb, Laura
Lt.(jg) Chapman, Mary Francis
Ens. Bertha Rae Evans
Lt.(jg) Gorzelanski, Helen Clara
Ens. Harrington, Mary Rose
Ens. Nash, Margaret Alice

Ens. O'Haver, Goldia Aimee
Ens. Paige, Eldene Elinor
Ens. Pitcher, Susie Josephine
Ens. Still, Dorothy
Ens. Todd, C. Edwina

U.S. Naval Hospital on Guam:**

Chief Nurse Lt.(jg) Olds, Marian
Ens. Christiansen, Lorraine
Ens. Fogarty, Virginia

Lt.(jg) Jackson, Leona
Ens. Yetter, Doris

---

* Biographical sketches, Record Group 52, National Archives, Washington, D.C.

** Lt. Comdr. Richard J. Bergren, USN, "Navy Nurse Corps WWII, A Complete Listing of Navy Nurses Held Prisoner of War by the Japanese During World War II," Bureau of Medicine and Surgery, U.S. Navy, Washington, D.C.

Appendix C

Military Nurses Who Were Not Reassigned following the Japanese Attack on the Philippines *

Nurses Assigned to Ft. Mills, Corregidor:

Chief Nurse 1st Lt. Mealer, Gladys

2d Lt. Anschicks, Louise M.

2d Lt. Black, Earlyn

2d Lt. Dworsky, Bertha H.

2d Lt. Eckman, Magdalina

2d Lt. Fails, Eula M.

2d Lt. Gardner, Helen L.

2d Lt. Garen, Eleanor M.

2d Lt. Greenwalt, Beulah M.

2d Lt. Madden Winifred P.

2d Lt. Stevens, Mabel V.

2d Lt. Stoltz, Ruth M.

2d Lt. Young, Eunice

Nurses Assigned to Camp John Hay, Baguio:

2d Lt. Bradley, Ruby G.

2d Lt. Chambers, Beatrice

---

* List is a compilation of information taken from Josephine Nesbit's "History of the Army Nurse Corps in the Philippine Islands," Washington, D.C., September 1940–February 1945 and information provided by the Department of Veterans Affairs.

Appendix D

Evacuation of U.S. Military Nurses from Manila, December 1941*

From Sternberg to Ft. Mills, Corregidor:

2d Lt. Aasen, Mina

2d Lt. Acorn, Catherine M.

2d Lt. Arnold, Phyllis

2d Lt. Burris, Myra V.

2d Lt. Dalton, Mildred

Capt. Davison, Maude

2d Lt. Hennessey, Helen

2d Lt. Henshaw, Gwendolyn L.

2d Lt. Hook, Willa

2d Lt. Lee, Harriet G.

2d Lt. Ludlow, Dorothy L.

Mrs. Kuehlthau, Brunetta A.[1]

Miss Motley, Ruby[2]

1st Lt. MacDonald, Florence.

2d Lt. McHale, Letha

2d Lt. McKay, Hortense

2d Lt. Nesbit, Josephine M.

1st Lt. O'Neill, Eleanor E.

2d Lt. Palmer, Rita G.

2d Lt. Peterson, Mollie A.

2d Lt. Putnam, Beulah M.

2d Lt. Straub, Ruth M.

2d Lt. Ullom, Madeline M.

---

* List is a compilation of information taken from Josephine Nesbit's "History of the Army Nurse Corps in the Philippine Islands," Washington, D.C., September 1940–February 1945 and information provided by the Department of Veteran Affairs.

[1] Physiotherapist commissioned in the U.S. Army as a medical specialist on 3 May 1944.

[2] Dietician commissioned in the U.S. Army as a medical specialist on 6 May 1944.

To Limay, Hospital No.1, Bataan:
Evacuated on 24 December 1941

2d Lt. Allen, Earleen

2d Lt. Barre, Agnes D.

Lt.(jg) Bernatitis, Ann

2d Lt. Corns, Edith M.

2d Lt. Easterling, Dorcas

2d Lt. Hogan, Rosemary

2d Lt. Gastinger, Leona

2d Lt. Gates, Marcia L.

2d Lt. Gillahan, Nancy J.

2d Lt. Hallman, Grace D.

2d Lt. Jenkins, Geneva

2d Lt. Jenkins, Ressa

2d Lt. Kennedy, Imogene

2d Lt. Lewey, Frankie T.

2d Lt. McDonald, Inez

2d Lt. Moultrie, Mary L.

2d Lt. Redmond, Juanita

2d Lt. Rieper, Rose E.

2d Lt. Summers, Helen

2d Lt. Veley, Beth A.

2d Lt. Whitlow, Evelyn B.

2d Lt. Wilson, Lucy

2d Lt. Wimbery, Edith M.

2d Lt. Wurts, Anne B.

2d Lt. Zwicker, Alice M.

Evacuated on 25 or 26 December 1941

2d Lt. Brantley, Hattie R.

2d Lt. Brown, Mary B.

2d Lt. Cassiani, Helen M.

2d Lt. Daley, Dorothea

2d Lt. Henson, Verna V.

2d Lt. Meyer, Adolpha

2d Lt. Scholl, Dorothy B.

To Hospital No.2, Bataan:

2d Lt. Bickford, Clara M.

2d Lt. Blaine, Ethel L.

2d Lt. Breese, Minnie

2d Lt. Dollason, Kathryn L.

2d Lt. Downing, Susan K.

2d Lt. Durrett, Sallie

2d Lt. Foreman, Adele F.

2d Lt. Hahn, Alice J.

2d Lt. Hahn, Alice J.

2d Lt. Kehoe, Doris

2d Lt. Kimball, Blanche

2d Lt. Lee, Eleanor O.

2d Lt. Lohr, Mary G.

To Hospital No.2, Bataan

2d Lt. Mueller, Clara

2d Lt. Nash, Frances[1]

2d Lt. Oberst, Mary

2d Lt. Reppak, Mary J.

2d Lt. Schacklette, Edith

2d Lt. Thor, Ethel M.

2d Lt. Williams, Anna E.

Mrs. Williams, Maude[2]

---

[1] Originally was assigned to this group, but was ordered to Hospital No.1 on 26 December 1941.

[2] Joined this group on 10 January 1942 and recommissioned in the U.S. Army Nurse Corps in 1942.

Appendix E

Evacuees from the Philippines to Australia

Aboard the Mactan, on 31 December 1941

2nd Lt. Floramund A. Fellmeth, ANC

Aboard two Navy PBYs, 29 April 1942[*]

PBY #1[**]

Crew:
Lt. Comdr. Edgar T. Neale, USN
Lt.(jg) Thomas F. Pollock, USN
D. W. Bounds, NAP, ACMM, USN
M. Ferrara, ACMM, USN, Plane captain
L. Gassett, ARM1c, USN, 1st radioman
W.F. Drexl, AMM1c, USN, 2d mech.
H.F. Donahue, ARM2c, USN, 2d radio

Passengers:

Brig. Gen. O. Seales, USA	Lt. J.C. Weschler, USN
Mrs. Seales	Lt. DeLong, USN (MTB)
Comdr. F.J. Bridgett, USN	Lt. Eileen Allen, ANC

---

[*] The passenger list is taken from Lt.(jg) Thomas Pollock, "Gridiron Flight: Narrative Report of Flight from Australia to Manila Bay and Return," p.6, Record Group 38, National Archives, Washington, D.C.
[**] PBY #1 was damaged and later repaired.

Lt. Lois Auschicks, ANC
Lt. Agnes Barre, ANC
Lt. Rosemary Hogan, ANC
Lt. Rita Palmer, ANC
Lt. Peggy O'Neil, ANC
Lt. Geneva Jenkins, ANC
Lt. Helen Gardiner, ANC
Lt. Sally Blaine, ANC
Lt. Whitlow, ANC
Mrs. Virginia Bradley, wife of
    army officer

Mrs. "Boots" Ryder, wife of
    navy officer
Lt. L.A. Erickson, AC
Lt. H.J. Dennison, AC
Lt. Col. of U.S. Army Finance
    Dept.
Two Filipino 2d lts.
Unidentified passengers

PBY #7

Crew:
Lt.(jg) L.C. Deede, A-V(N), USNR
Lt.(jg) William V. Gough, A-V(N), USNR
W. D. Eddy Nap, ACMM, USN
M. H. Crain, AMM1c, USN, plane captain
M. C. Lohr, AMM1c, USN 2d mech.
E. W. Bedford, ARM1c, USN, 1st radioman
W. F. Kelley, ARM3c, USN, 2d radioman

Passengers to Mindanao:
Lt. Col. W.W. Fertig, CE (later guerilla leader)
Maj. W.J. Latimer, OD
Maj. Jose Raxon, PA

Passengers picked up at Mindanao:
Capt. J.H.S. Dessez, USN   Lt. W. Cohen (MC) USN
Lt. Brantington, USN   Ens. J.A. Patterson, USNR

Passengers landed at Perth:
Comdr. C.H. Williams, USN   Mrs. Susan K. Downing
Comdr. W.W. Hastings, USN   Mrs. L.B. Beweley
Lt. T.K. Bowers, USN   Miss Virginia Beweley

Passengers landed at Darwin:

Maj. Wm. R. Bradford, AC	Lt. Juanita Redmond, ANC
Lt. Hugh H. Marble, AC	Lt. Harriet G. Lee, ANC
Lt. C.A. Allard, AC	Lt. Eunice O. Hatchitt, ANC
Lt. J.R. Griffin, AC	Lt. Willa L. Hook, ANC
Lt. Florence MacDonald, ANC	Lt. Catherine M. Acorn, ANC
Lt. Dorothea M. Daley, ANC	Father Edwin Ronan
Lt. Ressa Jenkins, ANC	Kall, ACOM, USN
Lt. Mary G. Lohr, ANC	1 soldier, U.S. Army

Aboard the submarine Spearfish, *3 May 1942**

U.S. Army Personnel:

Col. Charles Savage, AC	2d Lt. Grace Hallman, ANC
Col. Thomas Doyle, Inf.	2d Lt. Mary L. Moultrie, ANC
Col. Constant L. Irwin, GSC	2d Lt. Mollie A. Peterson, ANC
Col. Milton A. Hill, IGD	2d Lt. Ruth Straub, ANC
Col. Royal Jenks, FD	2d Lt. Mabel V. Stevens, ANC
Col. Mott Ramsey, VC	2d Lt. Helen Summers, ANC
2d Lt. Leona Gastinger, ANC	2d Lt. Beth Veley, ANC
2d Lt. Nancy Gillahan, ANC	2d Lt. Lucy Wilson, ANC
2d Lt. Hortense E. McKay, ANC	

U.S. Navy Personnel:

Comdr. R.G. Deewall
Comdr. E.L. Sackett
Comdr. H.C. Wilson (CEC)
Lt. Comdr. T.W. Davidson
Lt. Comdr. L.C. Parker
Lt. Comdr. D.W. Knoll

---

* List of names taken from "Allied Naval Forces Based Western Australia, Serial SA-115: USS *Spearfish* Special Mission: Forwards Narrative Account of Evacuation of Personnel from Corregidor, P.I. on 3 May 1942 During Fourth War Patrol," National Archives and Records Administration, Naval History Division, Washington, D.C., 3 June 1942, pp.1–2.

U.S. Navy Personnel:

Bill Scott, RM1c (unauthorized passenger)

Lt.(jg) Ann Bernatitis, NC

Civilians/Military Dependents:

Mrs. Margaret Janson, wife of naval officer

Chester Judah (unauthorized passenger-status unknown)

Appendix F

POW Army Nurses by Year of Birth (YOB), Age, Height, Weight at Captivity (WAC), Weight at Liberation (WAL), and Weight Loss*

Name	YOB	Age	Height	WAC	WAL	Loss
Aasen, Mina A	1894	51	5'6"	149	111	38
Anschicks, Louise	1892	53	5'0"	115	90	25
Arnold, Phyllis J.	1916	29	5'4"	120	100	20
Barre, Agnes	1912	33	NA	NA	NA	NA
Bickford, Clara M.	1917	28	5'7"	126	110	16
Black, Earlyn M.	1918	27	5'8"	140	123	17
Blaine, Ethel L.	1915	30	NA	NA	NA	NA
Bradley, Ruby G.	1907	38	5'4"	112	92	20
Brantley, Hattie R.	1916	29	5'7"	145	127	18
Breese, Minnie L.	1911	34	5'4"	123	107	16
Burris, Myra V.	1906	39	5'6"	150	125	25
Cassiani, Helen M.	1917	28	5'3"	176	117	59
Chambers, Beatrice	1910	34	5'5"	120	101	19
Corns, Edith M.	1913	32	5'6"	156	125	31
Dalton, Mildred J.	1914	31	5'6"	130	115	15
Davison, Maude C.	1885	60	5'2"	156	80	76

*Data taken from "Figures on Weight of Liberated Nurses," United States Army Nurse Corps Records, Washington, D.C., March 1945.

Name	YOB	Age	Height	WAC	WAL	Loss
Dollason, Kathyrn L.	1913	32	5'9"	130	110	20
Durrett, Sallie P.	1914	31	5'6"	125	115	10
Dworsky, Bertha H.	1910	35	5'5"	129	105	24
Easterling, Dorcas	1914	31	5'1"	120	96	24
Eckmann, Magdalina	1911	34	5'4"	145	125	20
Foreman, Adela F.	1912	33	5'3"	130	110	20
Francis, Earleen A.	1910	35	NA	135	97	38
Gardner, Helen L.	1914	31	5'4"	110	104	6
Garen, Eleanor M.	1909	36	5'5"	143	113	30
Gates, Marcia L.	1915	30	5'4"	124	108	16
Greenwalt, Beulah	1911	34	5'5"	128	108	20
Hahn, Alice J.	1917	28	5'8"	145	126	19
Hennessey, Helen	1913	32	5'4"	134	111	23
Henshaw, Gwen	1914	31	5'6"	135	103	32
Henson, Verna V.	1914	31	5'5"	117	92	25
Hogan, Rosemary	1915	30	5'9"	165	140	25
Jenkins, Geneva	1910	35	5'4"	134	100	34
Kehoe, Doris A.	1911	34	5'2"	123	105	18
Kennedy, Imogene	1918	27	NA	115	100	15
Kimball, Blanche	1921	24	5'5"	NA	NA	NA
Kuehlthau, Brunetta	1903	42	NA	140	102	38
Lee, Eleanor O.	1915	30	5'4"	NA	NA	NA
Lewey, Frankie T.	1910	35	5'5"	155	122	33
Ludlow, Dorothy L.	1916	29	5'5"	130	100	30
McDonald, Inez V.	1912	33	5'7"	122	110	12
McHale, Letha	1905	40	5'4"	100	68	32
Madden, Winifred	1911	34	5'3"	115	103	12
Mealer, Gladys N.	1904	41	5'3"	132	103	29
Meyer, Adolpha M.	1905	40	5'6"	160	98	62
Motley, Ruby F.	1906	39	NA	120	108	12
Mueller, Clara L.	1901	44	5'3"	128	97	31
Nash, Frances L.	1911	34	5'7"	140	118	22
Nesbit, Josephine	1894	51	5'7"	187	149	38
Oberst, Mary J.	1913	32	5'5"	125	115	10
O'Neill, Eleanor E.	1892	53	5'4"	142	98	44

Name	YOB	Age	Height	WAC	WAL	Loss
Palmer, Rita G.	1918	27	5'4"	120	85	35
Putnam, Beulah	1908	37	5'3"	155	115	40
Reppak, Mary J.	1914	31	5'4"	116	100	16
Rieper, Rose E.	1903	42	4'11"	125	74	51
Scholl, Dorothy B.	1913	32	5'6"	124	108	16
Schacklette, Edith	1908	37	5'3"	120	96	24
Stoltz, Ruth M.	1914	31	5'8"	130	110	20
Thor, Ethel M.	1910	35	5'5"	147	120	27
Ullom, Madeline M.	1911	34	5'2"	124	105	21
Weissblatt, Vivian	1905	40	NA	126	94	32
Whitlow, Evelyn B.	1916	29	5'5"	134	112	22
Williams, Anna E.	1917	28	5'6"	138	120	18
Williams, Maude D.	1907	38	NA	150	118	32
Wimberly, Edith M.	1911	34	5'4"	137	113	24
Wurts, Anne B.	1903	42	5'3"	113	92	21
Young, Eunice F.	1913	32	5'6"	125	110	15
Zwicker, Alice M.	1916	29	5'4"	120	105	15

Appendix G

POW Military Nurses by Year of Birth (YOB), Military Branch, Entered on Duty (EOD), Release Active Duty (RAD), Length of Service (LOS), and Highest Rank Attained*

[NA: (data) not available]

Name	YOB	Branch	EOD	RAD	LOS	Rank
Aasen, Mina A.	1894	Army	1918	1946	28	Capt.
Anschicks, Louise	1892	Army	1926	1946	20	Capt.
Arnold, Phyllis J.	1916	Army	1940	1946	5	1st Lt.
Barre, Agnes	1912	Army	1937	1948	11	NA
Bickford, Clara M.	1917	Army	NA	1945	NA	1st Lt.
Black, Earlyn M.	1918	Army	1940	1946	6	1st Lt.
Blaine, Ethel L.	1915	Army	1940	1947	6	NA
Bradley, Ruby G.	1907	Army	1934	1963	30	Col.
Brantley, Hattie R.	1916	Army	1939	1946		
(2 terms)			1954	1969	25	Lt. Col.
Breese, Minnie L.	1911	Army	NA	NA	NA	NA
Burris, Myra V.	1906	Army	1940	1946	5	1st Lt.
Cassiani, Helen M.	1917	Army	1941	1946	5	1st Lt.
Chambers, Beatrice	1910	Army	1940	1960	20	Maj.

---

*Compilation of information provided by the Department of Defense and the Department of Veterans Affairs, 1990.

Name	YOB	Branch	EOD	RAD	LOS	Rank
Chapman, Mary	1915	Navy	1936	NA	NA	NA
Cobb, Laura Mae	1892	Navy	1918	1947	29	Cmdr.
Corns, Edith M.	1913	Army	NA	NA	NA	NA
Dalton, Mildred J.	1914	Army	1939	1946	6	1st Lt.
Davison, Maude C.	1885	Army	1918	1946	27	Major
Dollason, Kathryn L.	1913	Army	1936	1958	22	NA
Durrett, Sallie P.	1914	Army	1937	1946	9	Capt.
Dworsky, Bertha H.	1910	Army	1940	1946	5	Capt.
Easterling, Dorcas	1914	Army	1940	1946		
(2 terms)			1946	1949	6	NA
Eckmann, Magdalena	1911	Army	NA	1946	NA	1st Lt.
Evans, Bertha Rae	1904	Navy	1931	1955	24	Capt.
Foreman, Adela F.	1912	Army	1941	1962	21	Major
Francis, Earleen A.	1910	Army	1938	1945	7	1st Lt.
Gardner, Helen L.	1914	Army	1939	1947	8	1st Lt.
Garen, Eleanor M.	1909	Army	1941	1959	18	Major
Gates, Marcia L.	1915	Army	NA	1946	NA	1st Lt.
Gorzelanski, Helen	NA	Navy	1935	NA	NA	NA
Greenwalt, Beulah	1911	Army	1937	1946	9	1st Lt.
Hahn, Alice J.	1917	Army	NA	1945	NA	1st Lt.
Harrington, Mary R.	NA	Navy	1937	NA	NA	NA
Hennessey, Helen	1913	Army	1940	1967	27	Lt. Col.
Henshaw, Gwen.	1914	Army	1936	1947	10	Capt.
Henson, Verna V.	1914	Army	1940	1946	6	1st Lt.
Hogan, Rosemary	1915	Army	1936	1962	25	Col.
Jenkins, Geneva	1910	Army	1941	1947	6	1st Lt.
Kehoe, Doris A.	1911	Army	NA	1963	20+	Col.
Kennedy, Imogene	1918	Army	1941	1946	5	1st Lt.
Kimball, Blanche	1921	Army	NA	1946	NA	1st Lt.
Kuehlthau, Brunetta	1903	Army	1944	1958	14	Major
Lee, Eleanor O.	1915	Army	1930	1947	18	NA
Lewey, Frankie T.	1910	Army	NA	1946	NA	1st Lt.
Ludlow, Dorothy L.	1916	Army	NA	1946	NA	Capt.
McDonald, Inez V.	1912	Army	NA	NA	NA	NA
McHale, Letha	1905	Army	NA	1946	NA	1st Lt.

Name	YOB	Branch	EOD	RAD	LOS	Rank
Madden, Winifred	1911	Army	1938	1961	23	Lt. Col.
Mealer, Gladys N.	1904	Army	1930	1946	15	Capt.
Meyer, Adolpha	1905	Army	NA	NA	NA	NA
Motley, Ruby F.	1906	Army	1944	1947	3	1st Lt.
Mueller, Clara L.	1901	Army	1932	1946	14	Capt.
Nash, Frances L.	1911	Army	1936	1950	15	Major
Nash, Margaret A.	1911	Navy	1936	1946	10	Lt. Cmdr.
Nesbit, Josephine M.	1894	Army	1918	1946	28	Maj.
Oberst, Mary J.	1913	Army	1937	1947	10	Capt.
O'Haver, Goldia A.	1902	Navy	1929	1946	17	Lt. Cmdr.
O'Neill, Eleanor E.	1892	Army	1919	1946	27	Capt.
Paige, Eldene E.	1913	Navy	1936	NA	NA	NA
Palmer, Rita G.	1918	Army	1941	1946	5	1st Lt.
Pitcher, Susie J.	1901	Navy	1929	1946	16	Lt. Cmdr.
Putnam, Beulah	1908	Army	1932	1946	14	1st Lt.
Reppak, Mary J.	1914	Army	NA	1960	20+	Maj.
Rieper, Rose E.	1903	Army	1937	1954	17	Maj.
Scholl, Dorothy B.	1913	Army	1940	1946	6	1st Lt.
Schacklette, Edith	1908	Army	1936	1957	21	Lt. Col.
Still, Dorothy	1914	Navy	1937	1947	9	Lt. Cmdr.
Stoltz, Ruth M.	1914	Army	NA	NA	NA	NA
Thor, Ethel M.	1910	Army	1938	1946	8	1st Lt.
Todd, Carrie Edwina	1911	Navy	1936	1966	30	Capt.
Ullom, Madeline M.	1911	Army	1938	1964	25	Lt. Col.
Weissblatt, Vivian	1905	Army	1942	1946	4	NA
Whitlow, Evelyn B.	1916	Army	1940	1946	6	1st Lt.
Williams, Anna E.	1917	Army	1940	1947	7	1st Lt.
Williams, Maude D.	1907	Army	1930	1939		
(3 terms)			1942	1945		
			1947	1969	23	Lt. Col.
Wimberly, Edith M.	1911	Army	1938	1958	20	Lt. Col.
Wurts, Anne B.	1903	Army	1941	1946	5	1st Lt.
Young, Eunice F.	1913	Army	1939	1961	22	Lt. Col.
Zwicker, Alice M.	1916	Army	NA	NA	NA	NA

Appendix H

Military Grades during World War II

Army Rank Abbreviations

2d Lt.: Second Lieutenant
1st Lt.: First Lieutenant
Capt.: Captain
Maj.: Major
Lt. Col.: Lieutenant Colonel
Col.: Colonel
Brig. Gen.: Brigadier General
Maj. Gen.: Major General
Lt. Gen.: Lieutenant General
Gen.: General

Navy Rank Abbreviations

Ens.: Ensign
Lt.(jg): Lieutenant Junior Grade
Lt.: Lieutenant
Lt. Comdr.: Lieutenant Commander
Comdr.: Commander
Capt.: Captain
Com. : Commodore
Rear Adm.: Rear Admiral
Vice Adm.: Vice Admiral
Adm.: Admiral

Notes

1. Pacific Paradise

1. Minnie Breese Stubbs, Department of Defense interview, Washington, D.C., 9 April 1983, p. 3.

2. Anna Eleanor Williams Clark, Department of Defense interview, Washington, D.C., 9 April 1983, p. 2.

3. Earlyn Black Harding, Department of Defense interview, Washington, D.C., April 1983, p. 2.

4. Clark interview, p. 4.

5. Lt. Col. Madeline Ullom, USA, NC (Ret.), interview with authors, Atlanta, Ga., 10 October 1991, p. 5.

6. Lt. Col. Hattie R. Brantley, USA, NC (Ret.), interview with authors, Atlanta, Georgia, March 1989.

7. Rita Palmer James, U.S. Army Nurse Corps Oral History Program interview, Stanley, Idaho, 5–6 June, 1984, p. 7.

8. Comdr. Edwina C. Todd, NC, USN, "Nursing Under Fire," *Military Surgeon* 100(Apr. 1947): 74.

9. Leona Jackson, RN, U.S. Navy Nurse Corps, "I Was on Guam," *American Journal of Nursing* 42(Nov. 1942): 1244–46.

10. Bertha Evans St. Pierre, Department of the Navy, Bureau of Medicine and Surgery interview, Orlando, Florida, 20 May 1992, pp. 4–5.

11. Phyllis Arnold Adams, U.S. Army Nurse Corps Oral History Program interview, Washington, D.C., April 1983, p. 4.

2. Paradise Lost

1. Maj. Josephine Nesbit Davis, USA, NC (Ret.), Department of Defense interview, Washington, D.C., April 1983, p. 2.

2. Col. Ruby Bradley, USA, NC (Ret.), U.S. Army Nurse Corps Oral History Program interview, Washington, D.C., 19 September 1984, pp. 7–8.

3. Ibid., p. 9.

4. Lt. Col. Hattie R. Brantley, USA, NC (Ret.), interview with authors, Atlanta, Georgia, March 1989, p. 3.

5. Phyllis Arnold Adams, U.S. Army Nurse Corps Oral History Program interview, Washington, D.C., April 1983, pp. 5–6.

6. Anna Eleanor Williams Clark, Department of Defense interview, Washington, D.C., 9 April 1983, pp. 7–8.

7. Ibid., p. 9.

8. Bertha Evans St. Pierre, Department of the Navy, Bureau of Medicine and Surgery interview, Orlando, Florida, 20 May 1992, p. 5.

9. Ibid.

10. "Last Message from Guam," *Army and Navy Journal,* 27 December 1941, p. 463.

11. "4 Navy Nurses Tell of Guam Capture on Arrival Here," Record Group 52, National Archives, Washington, D.C.

12. Leona Jackson, RN, U.S. Navy Nurse Corps, "I Was on Guam," *American Journal of Nursing* 42(Nov. 1942): 1244.

13. Comdr. C. Edwina Todd, NC, USN, "Nursing Under Fire," *Military Surgeon* 100(Apr. 1947): 75.

14. Dorothy Still Terrill, U.S. Army Nurse Corps Oral History Program interview, Washington, D.C., 9 April 1983, p. 7.

15. St. Pierre interview, p. 6.

16. Todd, "Nursing Under Fire," p. 75.

17. Lt. Col. Madeline Ullom, USA, NC (Ret.), interview with authors, Atlanta, Georgia, 29 April 1989, p. 4.

18. Ibid.

19. Bradley interview, pp. 9–10.

20. Ibid., p. 11.

21. Ibid., pp. 11–12.

22. Ibid., p. 12.

3. Descent into Hell

1. Lt. Col. Hattie R. Brantley, USA, NC (Ret.), interview with authors, Atlanta, Georgia, Mar. 1989, p. 6.

2. Frances L. Nash, "Georgia Nurse's Own Story . . . My Three Years in a Jap Prison Camp," *Atlanta Journal Magazine,* 15 April 1945, p. 6.

3. Ibid.

4. Beatrice Chambers, U.S. Army Nurse Corps Oral History Program interview, Washington, D.C., 1984, p. 7.

5. Ibid., pp. 5–6.

6. Frederic H. Stevens, *Santo Tomas Internment Camp*: Stratford House, 1946, pp. 317–18.

7. Lt. Col. Madeline Ullom, USA, NC (Ret.), interview with authors, Atlanta, Georgia, 29 April 1989, p. 8.

8. Maj. Josephine Nesbit Davis, USA, NC (Ret.), Department of Defense interview, Washington, D.C., Apr. 1983, pp. 2–3.

9. Comdr. C. Edwina Todd, NC, USN, "Nursing Under Fire," *Military Surgeon,* April 1947, p. 76.

10. Capt. Florence MacDonald, ANC, "Nursing the Sick and Wounded at Bataan and Corregidor," *Hospitals,* Dec. 1942, pp. 31–33.

11. Todd, "Nursing Under Fire," p. 76.

12. Ibid.

13. Ibid.

14. Ibid., p. 74.

4. The Other Alamo

1. Lt. Col. Hattie R. Brantley, ANC (Ret.), interview with authors, Atlanta, Georgia, Mar. 1989, p. 2.

2. Ibid.

3. Ibid., p. 3.

4. Bertha Dworsky Henderson, Department of Defense interview, Washington, D.C., April 1983, p. 4.

5. Gen. Jonathan M. Wainwright, *General Wainwright's Story* (Garden City, N.Y.: Doubleday, 1946), p. 45.

6. Alfred A. Weinstein, M.D., *Barbed-Wire Surgeon* (New York: Macmillan, 1947), p. 16.

7. Brantley interview, p. 5.

8. Maj. Josephine Nesbit Davis, USA, NC (Ret.), "Brief Autobiography of Major Josephine May Nesbit Davis," Washington, D.C., 2 April 1983, p. 2.

9. Maj. Josephine Nesbit Davis, USA, NC (Ret.), Department of Defense interview, Washington, D.C., 9 April 1983, p. 7.

10. Rita Palmer James, U.S. Army Nurse Corps Oral History Program interview, Stanley, Idaho, 5–6 June 1984, p. 61.

11. Davis interview, p. 8.

12. Weinstein, *Barbed-Wire Surgeon,* p. 33.

13. Lt. Col. William E. Dyess, *The Dyess Story* (New York: J.P. Putnam's Sons, 1944), p. 47.

14. Weinstein, *Barbed-Wire Surgeon,* p. 13.

15. Ibid., p. 27.

16. Wainwright, *General Wainwright's Story,* pp. 70–71.

17. Lt. Juanita Redmond, ANC, *I Served on Bataan* (Philadelphia: J.B. Lippincutt, 1943), p. 100.

18. Weinstein, *Barbed-Wire Surgeon,* p. 34.

19. Redmond, *I Served on Bataan,* p. 62.

20. Lt. Frances L. Nash, ANC, address to Grady Hospital staff, Atlanta, Ga., 1945, p. 3.

21. Ibid.

22. Redmond, *I Served on Bataan,* pp. 63–64.

23. Weinstein, *Barbed-Wire Surgeon,* p. 37.

24. Nash, address, p. 4.

25. Weinstein, *Barbed-Wire Surgeon,* p. 43.

26. Lt. Frances L. Nash, "Georgia Nurse's Own Story . . . My Three Years in a Jap Prison Camp," *Atlanta Journal Magazine,* 15 April 1945, p. 7.

27. Redmond, *I Served on Bataan,* p. 111.

28. James interview, p. 20.

29. Redmond, *I Served on Bataan,* pp. 114–15.

30. Nash, address, p. 4.

31. Davis, "Autobiography," p. 3.

5. From the Frying Pan into the Fire

1. Maude Denson Williams, *To the Angels* (San Francisco: Denson Press, 1984), pp. 76–77.

2. Lt. Col. Hattie R. Brantley, USA, NC (Ret.), interview with authors, Atlanta, Georgia, Mar. 1989, p. 9.

3. Lt. Hattie R. Brantley, USA, NC, "The Flight of the Army Nurses," *Ex-POW Bulletin 32* (Feb. 1975): 2.

4. Geneva Jenkins, Department of Defense interview, Washington, D.C., April 1983, pp. 8–9.

5. Frances L. Nash, "Georgia Nurse's Own Story . . . My Three Years in a Jap Prison Camp,"*Atlanta Journal Magazine,* 15 April 1945, p. 5.

6. Eric Morris, *Corregidor: The End of the Line* (New York: Stein and Day, 1984), p. 396.

7. Minnie Breese Stubbs, Department of Defense interview, Washington, D.C., April 1983, pp. 13–15.

8. Ibid.

6. The Tunnel and the Rock

1. Lt. Col. Hattie R. Brantley, USA, NC (Ret.), interview with authors, Atlanta, Georgia, Mar. 1989, p. 2.

2. Lt. Col. William E. Dyess, *The Dyess Story* (New York: J.P. Putnam's Sons, 1944), p. 26.

3. Helen Cassiani Nestor, Department of Defense interview, Washington, D.C., April 1983, p. 3.

4. Anna Eleanor Williams Clark, Department of Defense interview, Washington, D.C., 9 April 1983, p. 15.

5. Capt. Gladys Ann Mealer Giles, USA, NC (Ret.), Department of Defense interview, Washington, D.C., Apr. 1983, p. 1.

6. Lt. Col. Madeline Ullom, USA, NC (Ret.), Department of Defense interview, Washington, D.C., Apr. 9, 1983, p. 17.

7. Lt. Col. Madeline Ullom, USA, NC (Ret.), interview with authors, Atlanta, Georgia, 10 October 1991.

8. Lt. Juanita Redmond, ANC, *I Served on Bataan* (Philadelphia: J.B. Lippincutt, 1943), p. 142.

9. Lt. Frances L. Nash, address to Grady Memorial Hospital staff, Atlanta, Georgia, 1945, p. 2.

10. Ullom interview, pp. 15–16.

11. Minnie Breese Stubbs, Department of Defense interview, Washington, D.C., 1983, p. 16.

12. Capt. Thomas F. Pollock, USN (Ret.), "Operation Flight Gridiron," *Foundation Magazine,* Fall 1994, pp. 73–79.

13. Lt.(jg) Thomas F. Pollock, USN, "Gridiron Flight: Narrative Report of Flight from Australia to Manila Bay and Return," Record Group 38, National Archives, Washington, D.C., pp. 3–4.

14. Brantley interview, p. 18.

15. Pollock, "Gridiron Flight," pp. 8–9.

16. Ibid., p. 10.

17. Gen. Jonathan M. Wainwright, *General Wainwright's Story* (Garden City, N.Y.: Doubleday, 1946), p. 109.

18. Lucy Wilson Jopling, *Warrior in White* (San Antonio, Tex.: Watercress Press, 1990), p. 47, 50.

19. Ibid. p. 50.

20. Leona Gastinger Sutchin, interview with authors, Atlanta, Georgia, 29 April 1989, p. 23.

21. Wainwright, *General Wainwright's Story,* p. 110.

22. Brantley interview, p. 20.

23. Phyllis Arnold Adams, U.S. Army Nurse Corps Oral History Program interview, Washington, D.C., April 1983, p. 17.

24. Clark interview, pp. 19–20.

25. Verna Hively, Department of Defense interview, Washington, D.C., 9 April 1983, p. 6.

26. Giles interview, p. 18.

27. "Last Message from Corregidor," *Army and Navy Journal,* 6 June 1942, p. 1104.

28. Adams interview, pp. 17–18.

29. Frank A. Reister, *Medical Statistics in World War II* (Washington, D.C.: Department of the Army, Office of the Surgeon General, 1975), p. 44.

30. Giles interview, p. 19.

31. Brantley interview, p. 21.

32. Ullom Department of Defense interview, p. 20.

33. Ullom interview with authors, p. 20.

34. Ibid., p. 26.

35. Adams interview, p. 17.

36. Giles interview, pp. 20–21.

37. Stubbs interview, p. 18.

38. Giles interview, p. 22.

39. Ullom Department of Defense interview, p. 22.

7. The City of Hell

1. Lt. Col. Madeline Ullom, USA, NC (Ret.), interview with authors, Atlanta, Georgia, 29 April 1989, p. 9.

2. Lt. Col. Hattie R. Brantley, USA, NC (Ret.), interview with authors, Atlanta, Georgia, 9 May 1989, p. 6.

3. Ibid.

4. Rita Palmer James, U.S. Army Corps Oral History Program interview, Stanley, Idaho, 5–6 June 1984, p. 30.

5. Ullom interview, p. 11.

6. Anna Eleanor Williams Clark, Department of the Army interview, Sidney, Australia, 1 September 1983, pp. 2–3.

7. Ullom interview, p. 13.

8. Clark interview, pp. 2–3.

9. Brantley interview, p. 19.

10. Anna Eleanor Williams Clark, Department of Defense interview, Washington, D.C., 9 April 1983, p. 27.

11. Ibid., p. 3.

12. Lt. Col. Hattie R. Brantley, USA, NC (Ret.), Department of Defense interview, 9 April 1983, p. 28.

13. Reba Karp, "Her '66 Outlook Far Cry from That of '42," *Norfolk Virginian-Pilot* and *Portsmouth Star,* 16 January 1966.

14. Alice R. Clark, R.N., "Thirty-seven Months as Prisoner of War," *American Journal of Nursing,* 45 (May 1945), pp. 343

15. A.V.H. Hartendorp, *The Santo Tomas Story* (New York: McGraw-Hill, 1964), p. 100.

16. Lt. Eunice Young, ANC, diary, 1941–45, (San Francisco: Denson Press, 1984), p. 12.

17. Maude Denson Williams, *To the Angels* (San Francisco: Denson Press, 1984), pp. 159–60.

18. Hartendorp, *Santo Tomas Story,* p. 101.

8. Life along the River Styx

1. Capt. Gladys Ann Mealer Giles, USA, NC (Ret.), Department of Defense interview, Washington, D.C., April 1983, p. 26.

2. Lt. Eunice Young, ANC, diary, 1941–45, p. 14.

3. Ibid., p. 16.

4. Lt. Mary Jane Brown, NC, USNR, "The Joys of Meeting Pays the Pangs of Absence," *Trained Nurse and Hospital Review,* June 1945, pp. 411–12.

5. Young, diary, p. 17.

6. Lt. Col. Hattie R. Brantley, USA, NC (Ret.), Department of Defense interview, Washington, D.C., 9 April 1983, p. 28.

7. Maude Denson Williams, *To the Angels* (San Francisco: Denson Press, 1984), pp. 151–52.

8. Lt. Comdr. Laura Cobb, NC, USN, "Life in a Japanese Internment Camp," p. 4, Record Group 52, National Archives, Washington, D.C.

9. Ibid. pp. 4–5.

10. Williams, *To the Angels,* pp. 165–66.

11. Young, diary, p. 17.

12. Frederic H. Stevens, *Santo Tomas Internment Camp* (Stratford House, 1946), p. 414.

13. Young, diary, p. 18.

14. Anna Eleanor Williams Clark, Department of the Army interview, Sidney, Australia, 1 September 1983, pp. 2–3.

15. Col. Ruby Bradley, USA, NC (Ret.), Army Nurse Corps Oral History Program interview, Washington, D.C., 19 September 1984, p. 26.

16. Young, diary, p. 24.

17. Ibid., pp. 25–26.

18. Lt. Col. Madeline Ullom, USA, NC (Ret.), "A Santo Tomas Real Life Story," *Army Nurse,* Dec. 1974, p. 31, Eunice Young, "Angels of Bataan, Heroic Nurses of Bataan and Corregidor," American Ex-POWs, Inc., National Medical Research Committee Packet 20, p. 26.

19. Young, diary, p. 28.

20. Ibid.

21. Lt. Frances L. Nash, ANC, Address to Grady Hospital staff, Atlanta, Georgia, April 1945, p. 8.

22. A.V.H. Hartendorp, *The Santo Tomas Story* (New York: McGraw-Hill, 1964), pp. 200–201.

23. Young, diary, p. 30.

24. Ibid., p. 31.

9. Hunger in the Heart of Hell

1. Lt. Eunice Young, ANC, diary, 1941–45, pp. 33–34.

2. Earlyn Black Harding, Department of Defense interview, Washington, D.C., 9 April 1983, p. 18.

3. Young, diary, pp. 34–35.

4. Ibid., pp. 35–36.

5. Ibid., p. 35.

6. Lt. Col. Hattie R. Brantley, USA, NC (Ret.), interview with authors, Atlanta, Georgia, March 1989, p. 14.

7. Young, diary, p. 37.

8. *Prisoners of War Bulletin*, American Red Cross, Washington, D.C., June 1943, pp. 1–2.

9. Frances L. Nash, Address to Grady Hospital Staff, Atlanta, Georgia, 1945, p. 8.

10. Lt. Col. Madeline Ullom, USA, NC (Ret.), interview with authors, 29 April 1989, p. 21.

11. Lt. Col. Madeline Ullom, USA, NC (Ret.), interview with authors, 9 January 1998, p. 32.

12. A.V.H. Hartendorp, *The Santo Tomas Story* (New York: McGraw-Hill, 1964), p. 252.

13. Ullom interview, 9 January 1998, pp. 31–32.

14. Lt. Comdr. Laura M. Cobb, NC, USN, "Life in a Japanese Internment Camp," p. 5, Record Group 52, National Archives, Washington, D.C.

15. Comdr. C. Edwina Todd, NC, USN, "Nursing Under Fire," *Military Surgeon* 100 (April 1947): 78.

16. Ibid.

17. Young, diary, pp. 42–43.

18. Lt. Col. Madeline Ullom, USA, NC (Ret.), interview with authors, 10 October 1991, p. 22.

19. Beatrice E. Chambers, U.S. Army Nurse Corps Oral History Program interview, Washington, D.C., 1984, pp. 13–14.

20. Ibid.

21. Ibid., pp. 14–15.

22. Ibid., pp. 56–57.

23. Ibid., pp. 15–16.

24. Brantley interview, p. 18.

25. Ullom interview, 1998, p. 34.

26. Yuki Tanaka, *Hidden Horrors, Japanese War Crimes in World War II* (Boulder, Colo.: Westview Press, 1996), pp. 137–39.

27. Ibid., pp. 151–54.

28. Young, diary, pp. 43–44.

29. Ibid., p. 48.

30. Hartendorp, *Santo Tomas Story*, p. 300.

31. Ibid., p. 311.

32. Maj. Josephine Nesbit Davis, USA, NC (Ret.), letter to Dorothy Starbuck, Director of Veterans Benefits, Veterans Administration, Washington, D.C., 15 January 1983.

33. Young, diary, pp. 51–52.

34. Hartendorp, *Santo Tomas Story*, p. 329.

35. Young, diary, pp. 53–54.

36. Frederic Stevens, *Santo Tomas Internment Camp* (Stratford House, 1946), p. 161.

37. Lt. Col. Hattie R. Brantley, USA, NC (Ret.) interview with authors, Atlanta, Georgia, 9 May 1989, p. 21.

38. Ibid., p. 29.

39. Todd, "Nursing Under Fire," p. 80.

40. Ullom interview, 29 April 1989, p. 29.

41. Young, diary, pp. 60–61.

42. Anna Eleanor Williams Clark, Department of Defense interview, Washington, D.C., 9 April 1983, p. 27.

43. Frances L. Nash, "Georgia Nurse's Own Story . . . My Three Years in a Jap Prison Camp," *Atlanta Journal,* 22 April 1945, p. 6.

44. Stevens, *Santo Tomas Internment Camp*, p. 473.

45. Young, diary, p. 69.

46. Stevens, *Santo Tomas Internment Camp*, p. 475.

47. Ullom interview, 29 April 1989, p. 26.

48. Stevens, *Santo Tomas Internment Camp*, p. 478.

49. Young, diary, p. 73.

50. Ibid.

51. Ullom interview, 9 January 1998, p. 31.

52. Hartendorp, *Santo Tomas Story,* p. 403.

53. Stevens, *Santo Tomas Internment Camp,* p. 167.

10. Liberation

1. Minnie Breese Stubbs, Department of Defense interview, Washington, D.C., April 1983, p. 21.

2. Lt. Col. Madeline Ullom, USA, NC (Ret.), interview with authors, Atlanta, Georgia, 29 April 1989, p. 12.

3. Ibid., p. 30.

4. Ibid., p. 32.

5. Lt. Col. Hattie R. Brantley, USA, NC (Ret.), interview with authors, Atlanta, Georgia, 9 May 1989, p. 34.

6. A.V.H. Hartendorp, *The Santo Tomas Story* (New York: McGraw-Hill, 1964), p. 402.

7. Maude Denson Williams, *To the Angels* (San Francisco: Denson Press, 1984), p. 209.

8. Ibid., p. 210.

9. Ullom interview, p. 36.

10. Lt. Eunice Young, ANC, diary, 1941–45, p. 77.

11. Beatrice E. Chambers, U.S. Army Nurse Corps Oral History Program interview, Washington, D.C., 1984, pp. 20–21.

12. Ibid., p. 22.

13. Ibid., pp. 23–24.

14. Lt. Col. Maude Denson Williams, USAF (Ret.), interview with authors, Atlanta, Georgia, 1989, p. 39.

15. Young, diary, p. 78.

16. Williams interview, p. 39.

17. Helen Cassiani Nestor, Department of Defense interview, Washington, D.C., 9 April 1983, p. 25.

18. Maj. Josephine Nesbit Davis, USA, NC (Ret.), Department of Defense interview, Washington, D.C., 9 April 1983, p. 44.

19. Young, diary, pp. 82–83.

20. Ullom interview, p. 36.

21. Bertha Dworsky Henderson, Department of Defense interview, April 1983, p. 27.

22. Reba Karp, "Her '66 Outlook Far Cry from That of '42," *Norfolk Virginian-Pilot* and *Portsmouth Star,* 16 January 1966.

23. "Re: Death of George Louis," 28 January 1945, Record Group 52, National Archives, Washington, D.C.

24. Karp, "Her '66 Outlook Far Cry from That of '42."

25. Lt. Comdr. C. Edwina Todd, "Nursing Under Fire," *Military Surgeon* 100 (April 1947): 80.

26. Ibid.

27. Ibid., p. 81.

28. Laurie Johnston, "'We Want Waves' Is Shout of Liberated Navy Nurses, 'You Know, Permanent Waves,'" Honolulu, March 1945, Record Group 52, National Archives, Washington, D.C.

29. "25,000 Greet Lieut. Nash on Arrival Home," RG 52, National Archives, Washington, D.C.

30. "A Heroine Returns," RG 52, National Archives, Washington, D.C.

11. Home at Last

1. Minnie Breese Stubbs, Department of Defense interview, Washington, D.C., April 1983, p. 42.

2. Helen Cassiani Nestor, Department of Defense interview, Washington, D.C., 9 April 1983, pp. 11–12, 27.

3. Lt. Col. Hattie R. Brantley, USA, NC (Ret.), interview with authors, 5 July 1989, p. 34.

4. Stubbs interview, pp. 23–24.

5. Lt. Frances L. Nash, ANC, "Georgia Nurse's Own Story . . . My Three Years in a Jap Prison Camp," *Atlanta Journal Magazine,* 15 April 1945, p. 5.

6. Lt. Col. Madeline Ullom, USA, NC (Ret.), interview with authors, Atlanta, Georgia, 22 January 1998, p. 18.

7. Ibid., p. 14.

8. Ibid., p. 15.

9. Ibid., p. 16.

10. Rita Palmer James, U.S. Army Nurse Corps Oral History Program interview, Stanley, Idaho, 5–6 June 1984, p. 42.

11. Henderson interview, p. 29.

12. *Navy Women: A Pictorial History, 1908–1988,* vols.(Waves National, 1990), 1:15.

13. Lt. Col. Hattie R. Brantley, USA, NC (Ret.), interview with authors, Atlanta, Georgia, 5 February 1998, p. 3.

14. Lt. (jg) Leona Jackson, NC, USN, speech presented to navy personnel in Washington, D.C., 1942, p. 10, Department of the Navy, Bureau of Medicine and Surgery.

Bibliography

Adams, Phyllis Arnold. U.S. Army Nurse Corps Oral History Program interview, Washington, D.C., April 1983.

"Angels of Bataan: 68 Heroine Nurses Honored at Letterman." *San Francisco Chronicle*, 27 February 1945.

Army and Navy Joint News Release, Record Group 52, National Archives, Washington, D.C.

"Army Nurse Corps." *Army and Navy Journal*, 27 December 1941–30 May 1942.

"Army Nurses Liberated from Manila Internment Camp." *New York Times*, 22 February 1945.

Archard, Theresa. *G.I. Nightingale: The Story of an American Army Nurse.* New York: Norton, 1945.

"Bataan Wounded at Australia." *Army and Navy Journal*, 31 January 1942, p. 638.

Biographical Sketch: Lt.(jg) Laura M. Cobb, NC, USN, Record Group 52, National Archives, Washington, D.C.

Bradley, Col. Ruby, USA, NC (Ret.). U.S. Army Nurse Corps Oral History Program interview, Washington, D.C., 19 September 1984.

Brantley, Lt. Col. Hattie R., USA, NC (Ret.). Department of Defense interview, Washington, D.C., 9 April 1983.

———. "The Flight of the Army Nurses." *Ex-POW Bulletin* 32, (February 1975): 2–5.

———. Interviews with authors, Atlanta, Georgia, March 1989, 9 May 1989, 5 July 1989, 5 February 1998.

Brown, Lt. Mary Jane, NC, USNR. "The Joys of Meeting Pays the Pangs of Absence." *Trained Nurse and Hospital Review,* June 1945, pp. 411–12.

Butler, Allen, Julian Ruffin, Marion Sniffen et al. "The Nutritional Status of Civilians Rescued from Japanese Prison Camps." *New England Journal of Medicine* 233 (29 November 1945): 639–52.

Chambers, Beatrice E. U.S. Army Nurse Corps Oral History Program interview, Washington, D.C., 1984.

Clark, Alice R., RN. "Thirty-seven Months as Prisoners of War." *American Journal of Nursing* 45, (May 1945): 342–45.

Clark, Anna Eleanor Williams. Department of Defense interview, Washington, D.C., 9 April 1983.

———. Department of the Army interview, Sidney, Australia, 1 September 1983.

Cobb, Lt. Comdr. Laura NC, USN. "Life in a Japanese Internment Camp." Record Group 52, National Archives, Washington, D.C.

———. Outline. Record Group 52, National Archives, Washington, D.C.

Cooper, Page. *Navy Nurse.* New York: McGraw-Hill, 1946.

Cry Havoc. Film, MGM, Hollywood, California, 1943.

Danner, Dorothy Still. "Reminiscences of a Nurse POW." *Navy Medicine,* May–June 1992, pp. 36–40.

Davis, Dorothy. "I Nursed at Santo Tomas." *American Journal of Nursing* 44 (January 1944): 29–30.

———. "Nursing in Prison Camps." *Military Surgeon* 100 (January 1947): 42–46.

———. *The Road Back.* Lubbock: Texas Tech University Press, 1996.

Davis, Maj. Josephine Nesbit, USA, NC (Ret.). "Brief Autobiography of Major Josephine May Nesbit Davis." Washington, D.C., 2 April 1983.

———. Department of Defense interview, Washington, D.C., 9 April 1983.

———. Letter to Dorothy Starbuck, Director of Veterans Benefits, Veterans Administration, Washington, D.C., 15 January 1983.

Department of the Navy, Bureau of Medicine and Surgery. Washington, D.C., February–March 1998.

"Dispatches from Corregidor." *Army and Navy Journal,* 2 May 1942, p. 968.

Dyess, Lt. Col. William E. *The Dyess Story.* New York: G.P. Putnam's Sons, 1944.

"Eleven Navy and Three Civilian Nurses to Receive Bronze Star Medals for Work in Philippines." Record Group 52, National Archives, Washington, D.C.

"Eleven Navy Nurses Return After Three Years of Imprisonment." Record Group 52, National Archives, Washington, D.C.

Evans, Jessie Fant. "Nurse, Ex-Prisoner of Japs, Hopes to Return to Guam." Record Group 52, National Archives, Washington, D.C.

"Fall of Corregidor." *Army and Navy Journal*, 9 May 1942, p. 1009.

Farmer, Sallie Durrett. U.S. Army Nurse Corps Oral History Program interview, Washington, D.C., 15 May 1984.

"Figures on Weight of Liberated Nurses." U.S. Army Nurse Corps, March 1945. Record Group 52, National Archives, Washington, D.C.

"First Picture by Radio from Belgian Congo." Record Group 52, National Archives, Washington, D.C.

Flanagan, Lt. Gen. Edward M., USA (Ret.). *The Los Baños Raid: The 11th Airborne Jumps at Dawn.* Novato, Calif.: Presidio Press, 1986.

"Former Jap Prisoner Commends Red Cross." *The Seagull, Clearfield for the Personnel of the Naval Supply Depot at Clearfield, Utah,* 3 March 1945.

"4 Navy Nurses Tell of Guam Capture on Arrival Here." Record Group 52, National Archives, Washington, D.C.

Geister, Janet M., RN. "She Came Back from Bataan." *Trained Nurse,* October 1942, pp. 252–54.

Giles, Capt. Gladys Ann Mealer, USA, NC (Ret.). Department of Defense interview, Washington, D.C., April 1983.

Harding, Earlyn Black. Department of Defense interview, Washington, D.C., 9 April 1983.

Hartendorp, A.V.H. *The Santo Tomas Story.* New York: McGraw-Hill, 1964.

Haynes, Lt. Col. Edith Shacklette, USA, NC (Ret.). U.S. Army Nurse Corps Oral History Program interview, Washington, D.C., 9 April 1983.

Henderson, Bertha Dworsky. Department of Defense interview, Washington, D.C., April 1983.

Herman, Jan K. *Battle Station Sick Bay.* Annapolis, Md.: Naval Institute Press, 1997.

"The Heroic Nurses of Bataan and Corregidor." *American Journal of Nursing* 42 (August 1942): 896–98.

"A Heroine Returns." Record Group 52, National Archives, Washington, D.C.

Hibbs, Ralph E. "Beriberi in Japanese Prison Camp." *Annals of Internal Medicine* 45 (August 1946): 270–82.

Highlights in the History of the Army Nurse Corps. Washington, D.C.: U.S. Center for Military History, 1987.

Hively, Verna. Department of Defense interview, Washington, D.C., 9 April 1983.

Jackson, R.N., U.S. Navy Nurse Corps., Leona. "I Was on Guam." *American Journal of Nursing* 42 (November 1942): 1244–46.

———. Speech Presented to Navy Personnel in Washington, D.C., 1942. Department of the Navy, Bureau of Medicine and Surgery, Washington, D.C.

———. U.S. Naval Institute interview, Arlington, Virginia, 26 September 1986.

James, Rita Palmer. U.S. Army Nurse Corps Oral History Program interview, Stanley, Idaho, 5–6 June 1984.

Jenkins, Geneva. Department of Defense interview, Washington, D.C., April 1983.

Johnston, Laurie. "'We Want Waves,' Is Shout of 11 Liberated Navy Nurses, 'You Know, Permanent Waves.'" Honolulu, March 1945, Record Group 52, National Archives, Washington, D.C.

Johnston, Richard W. "68 'Angels of Bataan' Fly Back to Heaven After 3 Years of Prison Camp Hell." *Salt Lake City Tribune*, 25 February 1945.

Jopling, Lucy Wilson. *Warriors in White*. San Antonio, Tex.: Watercress Press, 1990.

Kalish, Philip A., and Beatrice Kalish. "Nurses Under Fire: The World War II Experience of Nurses of Bataan and Corregidor." *Nursing Research* 25 (November–December 1976): 409–29.

Karp, Reba. "Her '66 Outlook Far Cry From That of '42," *Norfolk Virginia–Pilot and Portsmouth Star*, 16 January 1966.

Kerr, E. Bartlett. *Surrender and Survival*. New York: William Morrow, 1985.

"Last Message from Corregidor." *Army and Navy Journal*, 6 June 1942, p. 1104.

"Last Message from Guam." *Army and Navy Journal*, 27 December 1941, p. 463.

Lloyd, Edith Corns. U.S. Army Oral History Program questionnaire, Washington, D.C., 1985.

MacDonald, Capt. Florence, ANC. "Nursing the Sick and Wounded at Bataan and Corregidor." *Hospitals*, December 1942, pp. 31–33.

Manchester, William. *American Caesar.* New York: Dell, 1978.

Matloff, Maurice, ed. *American Military History.* Washington, D.C.: Center of Military History, 1985.

Morris, Eric. *Corregidor: The End of the Line.* New York: Stein and Day, 1984.

Motley, 1st Lt. Ruby, M.D.D., A.U.S. "Bataan and Its Aftermath." *Journal of the American Dietetic Association* 22 (March 1946): 201–205.

Nash, Frances L. Address to Grady Hospital staff, Atlanta, Georgia, April 1945.

——. "Georgia Nurse's Own Story... My Three Years in a Jap Prison Camp." *Atlanta Journal Magazine,* 15 and 22 April 1945.

Nash, Lt. Margaret, NC, USN. "This Is My America." *True Confessions,* August 1945, p. 27.

"Navy Nurse Prisoners of War in Philippines." Record Group 52, National Archives, Washington, D.C.

"Navy Nurses Administer While Interned in P.I." Record Group 52, National Archives, Washington, D.C.

Navy Women: A Pictorial History, 1908–1988. Waves National, Vol. 1, 1990.

Nesbit, Major Josephine, USA, NC (Ret.). "Brief Autobiography of Major Josephine May Nesbit Davis," Washington, D.C., 9 April 1983.

——. Department of Defense interview, Washington, D.C., April 1983.

——. "History of the Army Nurse Corps in the Philippine Islands." Washington, D.C., September 1940–February 1945.

Nestor, Helen Cassiani. Department of Defense interview, Washington, D.C., 9 April 1983.

"Nursing on Bataan." *Pacific Coast Journal of Nursing,* July 1942, pp. 398–401.

Olds, Marion, Chief Nurse, U.S. Navy. "I Was a Prisoner at Guam." Speech at George Washington University Alumni Association, Record Group 52, National Archives, Washington, D.C.

"Pay of Missing Personnel." *Army and Navy Journal,* 7 February 1942, p. 664.

Pearson, Lt. Col. Emmet F. "Morbidity and Mortality in Santo Tomas Internment Camp." *Annals of Internal Medicine,* 24 (June 1946): 988–1002.

Pollock, Lt.(jg) Thomas F. "Gridiron Flight: Narrative Report of Flight from Australia to Manila Bay and Return." Record Group: 38, National Archives, Washington, D.C.

————. "Operation Flight Gridiron." *Foundation Magazine*. Fall 1994, pp. 73–79.

"Prisoners of War." *Army and Navy Journal*, 21 February 1942, pp. 682–84.

Prisoners of War Bulletin. American Red Cross, Washington, D.C., Vols. 1–3, 1943–45.

"Prisoners of War in Japan." *Army and Navy Journal*, 11 April 1942, p. 886.

"Re: Death of George Louis." 28 January 1945, Record Group 52, National Archives, Washington, D.C.

Redmond, Lt. Juanita, ANC. *I Served on Bataan*. Philadelphia: J.B. Lippincott, 1943.

Reister, Frank A. *Medical Statistics in World War II*. Washington, D.C.: Department of the Army, Office of the Surgeon General, 1975.

Romulo, Col. Carlos P. *I Saw the Fall of the Philippines*. New York: Doubleday, Doran, 1942.

So Proudly We Hail. Film, Paramount Pictures, Hollywood, Calif., 1943.

St. Pierre, Bertha Evans. Department of the Navy, Bureau of Medicine and Surgery interview, Orlando, Florida, 20 May 1992.

Stevens, Frederic H. *Santo Tomas Internment Camp*. Stratford House, 1946.

Stubbs, Minnie Breese. Department of Defense interview, Washington, D.C., April 1983.

Sutchin, Leona Gastinger. Interview with authors, Atlanta, Georgia, 29 April 1989.

Tanaka, Yuki. *Hidden Horrors: Japanese War Crimes in World War II*. Boulder, Colo.: Westview Press, 1996.

"Tells of Bataan." *Army and Navy Journal*, 18 April 1942, p. 902.

Terrill, Dorothy Still. U.S. Army Nurse Corps Oral History Program interview, Washington, D.C., 9 April 1983.

Todd, Comdr. C. Edwina, NC, USN. "Nursing Under Fire." *Military Surgeon* 100, (April 1947): 74–80.

Toland, John. *The Rising Sun: The Decline and Fall of the Japanese Empire, 1936–1945*. New York: Random House, 1970.

"25,000 Greet Lieut. Nash on Arrival Home." Record Group 52, National Archives, Washington, D.C.

Ullom, Lt. Col. Madeline, USA, NC (Ret.). Congressional Testimony before the U.S. Senate Veterans Affairs Committee, Phoenix, Ariz., 26 January 1982.

———. Department of Defense interview. Washington , D.C., 9 April 1983.

———. Interviews with authors, Atlanta, Georgia, 29 April 1989, 10 October 1991, 9 January 1998, 22 January 1998.

———. "Major Maude C. Davison, ANC." Tucson, Arizona, 29 October 1991.

———. "A Santo Tomas Real Life Story." *Army Nurse,* December 1974, pp. 29–34.

"U.S. War Communiques." *Army and Navy Journal,* 10 January–9 May 1942.

Valentine, Carolyn, B.S. "Nursing at Los Baños: Navy Nurses as Prisoners of War." *R.N.,* May 1945, pp. 30–68.

Wainwright, Gen. Jonathan M. *General Wainwright's Story.* Garden City, N.Y.: Doubleday, 1946.

"The War Program: Navy and Marines on Bataan." *Army and Navy Journal,* 11 April 1942, pp. 890–92.

We All Came Home. Video, Veterans Administration/Department of Defense, Washington, D.C., 1986.

Weinstein, Alfred A., M.D. *Barbed-Wire Surgeon.* New York: MacMillan, 1947.

Whittier, Roxane. "She Was a Prisoner of the Japs." Record Group 52, National Archives, Washington, D.C.

Williams, Maude Denson. Interview with authors, Atlanta, Georgia, 1989.

———. *To the Angels.* San Francisco: Denson Press, 1984.

Willenz, June A. *Women Veterans, America's Forgotten Heroines.* New York: Continuum, 1983.

Women of Valor. Movie for television, Hollywood, Calif., 1986.

Young, Eunice. "Angels of Bataan, Heroic Nurses of Bataan and Corregidor." American Ex-POWs, Inc., National Medical Research Committee Packet 20, p. 26.

———. Department of Defense interview, Washington, D.C., 9 April 1983.

———. Diary, 1941–45.

———. Interview with authors, Atlanta, Georgia, 29 April 1989.

———. "Three Years Outside This World." *Saturday Evening Post,* 5 May 1945, pp. 18-19, 89-90, 92.

Index

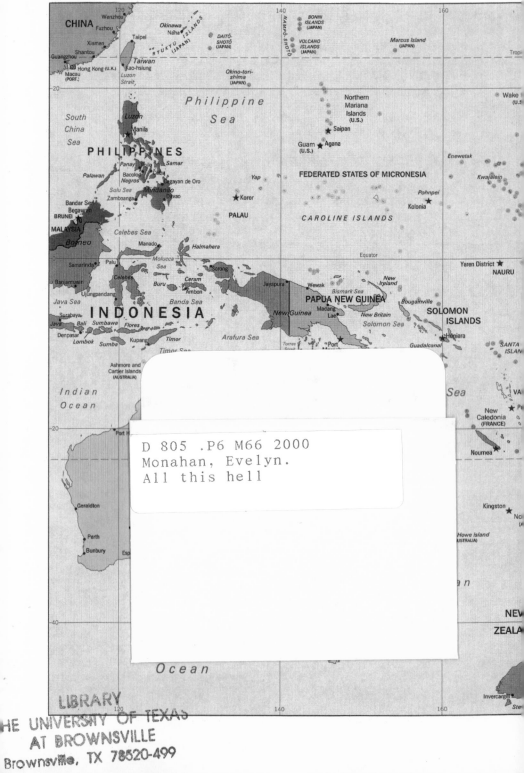

Oceania

CHINA

Wenzhou
Fuzhou
Xiamen
Shantou
Guangzhou
Hong Kong (U.K.)
Macau
(PORT.)

Okinawa
Naha

RYUKYU ISLANDS (JAPAN)

Taipei

Taiwan
Kao-hsiung
Luzon
Strait

*DAITŌ-
SHOTŌ
(JAPAN)*

NAMPO-SHOTŌ

BONIN
ISLANDS
(JAPAN)

VOLCANO
ISLANDS
(JAPAN)

Marcus Island
(JAPAN)

Tropi

Okino-tori-
shima
(JAPAN)

Wake
(U.S

South
China
Sea

Luzon

*Philippine
Sea*

Manila

Northern
Mariana
Islands
(U.S.)

★ Saipan

PHILIPPINES

Panay
Iloilo
Cebu
Samar

Palawan
Bacolod
Negros
Cagayan de Oro
Davao

Mindanao

Sulu Sea
Zamboanga

Bandar Seri
Begawan
BRUNEI
MALAYSIA

Borneo

Samarinda

Banjarmasin

Java Sea

Surabaya
Java
Bali
Sumbawa
Flores
Denpasar
Lombok
Sumba
Kupang

Ashmore and
Cartier Islands
(AUSTRALIA)

*Indian
Ocean*

Celebes Sea

Manado

Palu
Celebes

Ujungpandang

Guam ★ Agana
(U.S.)

Yap

★ Koror

PALAU

Enewetak

FEDERATED STATES OF MICRONESIA

Kwajalein

Pohnpei
Kolonia ★

CAROLINE ISLANDS

Halmahera

Molucca
Sea

Sorong

Ceram

Ambon
Buru

Banda Sea

Timor

Arafura Sea

Equator

Jayapura

Yaren District ★
NAURU

Wewak

Bismark Sea

New
Ireland

Madang
New Guinea
Lae

PAPUA NEW GUINEA

Bougainville

Solomon Sea

New Britain

SOLOMON
ISLANDS

Honiara

Guadalcanal

SANTA
ISLAN

Port H

Torres
Strait

Port

Geraldton

Perth
Bunbury
Esp

Ocean

Sea

New
Caledonia
(FRANCE)

Noumea

VA
★ Po

Kingston

No
(A

Howe Island
(AUSTRALIA)

n

NEW
ZEALA

Invercargill
Ste

120   140   160